The Momhak Method

The Empowered Path to Addiction Recovery: Master Your Mind & Body for Lasting Freedom

Rewire your mind. Reset your body. Reclaim your life.

By Pat McCashin

To my brother, Casey.
Forever in my heart, forever my inspiration.
And to everyone struggling with addiction:
These tools transformed my life. May they transform yours, too.

For permissions and inquiries:

pat@momhak.com | www.momhak.com

Cover design and interior layout by Pat McCashin

First Edition, 2025

ISBN (Paperback): 978-1-0694580-0-1

ISBN (eBook): 978-1-0694580-1-8

Published by Green Spring Research Publishing, Canada

Printed in the country of distribution

IMPORTANT DISCLAIMER

I am not a physician, therapist, or licensed medical professional, and this book is not intended as a substitute for professional counseling or medical advice. The practices covered within this book (including cold exposure, breathwork, and movement-based techniques) may carry risks. If you have a heart condition, respiratory issues, mental health challenges, or other medical concerns, please consult a qualified healthcare provider before trying these methods. Always listen to your body and use common sense. The author and publisher disclaim any liability for injuries or damages arising from the use or misuse of the techniques or advice contained in this book.

If you've been drinking heavily, abrupt withdrawal can be dangerous. Some stories here describe severe detox. If you suspect you need medical supervision, please consult a professional before stopping alcohol suddenly.

Names and identifying details of some of the people portrayed and/or quoted in this book have been changed.

INTRODUCTION

"You have power over your mind—not outside events. Realize this, and you will find strength."
—Marcus Aurelius

Let's see if any of this sounds familiar.

You've tried quitting, only to find yourself trapped in the same cycle.

You've sworn off a destructive habit, promising yourself that "this is the last time." Your willpower feels strong in the morning but crumbles by nightfall.

You've white-knuckled through cravings or felt frustrated that sheer determination isn't enough.

If all—or any—of the above strikes a chord, you're most definitely not alone. Many of us have been there, wondering why change feels so difficult, even when we desperately want it. The truth often isn't a lack of desire or a personal failing—it lies deeper, in the way destructive habits can subtly rewire our brain's reward system. Addiction and ingrained habits aren't about conscious choice; these things hijack our neurochemistry, making willpower an exhausting, and often losing, battle. When the brain itself is working against you, simply trying harder rarely leads to lasting freedom.

But what if there was a different way? What if, instead of fighting your urges head-on, you could systematically *rewire* the circuits driving them? This book unveils **The Momhak Method**: a unique, science-backed approach designed to do exactly that. It blends practical, body-based techniques like mindful movement and breathwork with powerful mind-hacking tools to help you reset your brain and reclaim control from the inside out. This isn't about surrendering—it's about harnessing your inherent capacity to change by working with your brain's natural ability to adapt.

A Different Path to Freedom

For me, the profound need for such a different path became undeniable a few years ago, on a quiet morning when I watched my brother, Casey, take his last breath, his body ravaged by decades of alcohol abuse. That moment changed *everything*—not just because I lost him, but because in his struggle, I saw the reflection of my own future if I didn't break the cycle.

While meetings and 12-step programs work for some of us, they definitely aren't the only path. I realized that lasting freedom required more than external support or sheer determination alone—it required tools to fundamentally change my internal landscape. Casey's story, and my own journey through repeated attempts to quit, forced me to look beyond conventional methods and explore ways to directly influence the brain and nervous system. This approach isn't for everyone—but if you're seeking a proactive, self-empowered route, it just might be exactly what you've been seeking.

Who This Book Is For

These chapters and the wisdom within them are for you if you're tired of conventional recovery approaches that don't quite fit, or if you've tried sheer willpower and traditional meetings without lasting results. Essentially, it's for anyone craving a more dynamic, hands-on method—a blend of practical movement, breathwork, and science-backed mind-rewiring.

It'll be especially helpful for those who believe in their own inner capacity for change and reject the notion of powerlessness. If you sense that meaningful recovery comes from harnessing your inherent strengths rather than surrendering to a higher power, you'll find that these teachings align with your perspective. The Momhak Method recognizes that you already have the power within you—you just need effective tools to activate it. This is true of anyone struggling with addiction, whether you're:

- A busy parent juggling real-life stress who needs a practical, effective approach to self-care
- A professional who can't afford another day lost to hangovers or low energy
- Someone who's struggled with moderation and is looking for a sustainable way forward
- A person who doesn't identify as an "addict" but senses that a habit is trying to take control
- Seeking a recovery method that isn't tied to group meetings or traditional 12-step models

Even if you don't identify with a specific "addiction" but sense a destructive habit creeping into your life, The Momhak Method provides tools to reclaim control, restore vitality, and design a future you love.

Why Willpower Wasn't Enough

Like you, I'd tried everything. Willpower. Meetings. White-knuckling through cravings that felt like they'd tear me apart. Sometimes I'd make it a few weeks or months, but I always found myself back in the same destructive patterns. **Why?** Because I hadn't changed the way my brain worked. The cravings, the stress, the need to escape… they were all still there, just waiting for a moment of weakness. I remember one morning particularly well—a moment that crystallized everything that wasn't working.

The Morning After: Facing the Truth

I woke up in a haze of sweat and regret, my head pounding like a war drum. The stale stench of alcohol and sweat clung to me, and my mouth was as dry as sandpaper. I could still taste the night before—bitter, sour, full of remorse. I checked my phone with dread, bracing for missed calls, angry messages, or maybe some humiliating memory lurking in my inbox.

But even worse than not knowing what I'd done was the sickening certainty that it had happened again.

Sitting up too fast and with nausea twisting my guts, I felt a pulse of blind rage. At what? At *myself*. At this cycle I swore I'd break. At the weak version of me, staring back in the mirror with puffy face and bloodshot eyes.

I clenched my fists. *Why am I like this? Why can't I stop?* Again and again, I'd sworn that it was the last time. I'd told myself that I could control it, that I just needed more willpower. Deep down, though, I knew the truth. **Willpower wasn't enough**.

Something had to change. *I* had to change. But how? The answer began to emerge not in a moment of crisis but instead in the quiet rhythms of my daily work.

How The Momhak Method Was Born

It didn't come to me in a moment of deep meditation or grand revelation—the name "The Momhak Method" arrived while I was doing my job as an archaeologist, surveying the forest. My work sometimes involves walking through forestry cut blocks before they're harvested, searching for signs of cultural heritage—First Nations village sites, culturally modified trees, or ancient campsites that need to be preserved.

On the surface, it's a job of observation, but I turned it into something more. As I moved through the woods, I practiced a form of **Moving Meditation**—syncing my breath with each step, staying aware of my movements, and scanning the trees for patterns that revealed the past. Sometimes, I'd weave in affirmations as I walked, subtly reprogramming my mind with each inhalation and exhalation.

And then it hit me like a bullet: The foundation of everything that was working for my sobriety boiled down to two principles:

1. **Moving Meditation:** Syncing breath and body—through Tai Chi, yoga, hiking, gardening, or any mindful movement.
2. **Mind Hacking:** Affirmations, cognitive reframing, cold exposure, breathwork (like the Wim Hof Method or 4–6 breathing) to shift the nervous system from fight-or-flight to calm, clear-headed balance.

Everything I'd learned about rewiring my brain, breaking addictive patterns, and reclaiming my life distilled into those two concepts: Moving Meditation and Mind Hacking—which together formed The Momhak Method.

How to Rewire Your Brain & Escape the Cycle

Lasting freedom from addiction isn't about willpower or meetings—it's about **rewiring your brain's reward system** using movement, breath, and strategic mindset shifts.

I looked deeper into neuroplasticity, cold exposure, breathwork, and moving meditation. As I watched my brother's struggle and my own repeated failures, I realized that addiction isn't just a battle of willpower—it's a battle of *wiring*. If I wanted lasting change, I had to stop fighting my brain and start **reprogramming** it at the source.

When I first tried these techniques, I wasn't sure they'd work, but within weeks, my cravings lessened, my mind felt clearer, and I handled stress better. I wasn't relying on willpower—I was **reshaping** my brain.

Ancient traditions have taught for centuries that we can reform our neural pathways, and modern research affirms it. Studies show that breathwork and Moving Meditation can strengthen self-control while reducing stress (Tang & Posner, 2015; see full reference in the Appendix C: Notes section). The Momhak Method blends these core principles into a practical, step-by-step system. More than traditional recovery, it's **mental reprogramming**, resetting your experience of pleasure, stress, and motivation.

This is the core of The Momhak Method. And the best part? You don't need to wait until you finish this book to begin experiencing its effects—in fact, you can take your first step in the next 60 seconds.

> *"The beginning is the most important part of the work."*
> —Plato

Your First Small Step—Right Now

Pause for a moment. Take a deep breath in for 4 seconds, then exhale slowly for 6 seconds. Now ask yourself: *What's the one thing I hope to change most by the time I finish this book?* Whisper the answer to yourself, write it down, or simply hold it in your mind. That intention is your first step toward transformation. But transformation doesn't happen in theory—it happens in action. For the next 30 days, take one small daily step, such as:

- Practicing 4–6 breathing when stress hits

- Switching to a refreshing burst of cold water in the middle of your shower

- Repeating an affirmation that resonates with you (e.g., "I'm relaxed, confident, and content thriving in sobriety.")

If you're ready, start today: Take another deep breath in for 4 seconds, and then exhale for 6. You've already begun. That one small action exemplifies what sets this approach apart from conventional recovery methods.

What Makes The Momhak Method Different?

While many programs focus on abstinence and accountability, **The Momhak Method** emphasizes building a life that's worth staying sober for, while at the same time transforming your mental state from the inside out. Here's why it stands apart:

- **Evidence-Informed Approach**
  Each practice is grounded in real-world research, from the neuroplasticity of affirmations to the dopamine boosts of Cold Exposure.

- **Personal Empowerment**
  We don't label you as "powerless." Instead, we highlight your brain's innate capacity to adapt. You can reclaim control because you're built for transformation.

- **Flexibility**
  There's no one-size-fits-all. Pick from a toolbox—from early riser to night owl, or seasoned athlete to physical activity rookie.

- **Integration**
  Physical practices, mental exercises, and emotional healing work together for lasting change. This synergy is the heart of The Momhak Method's success.

Science Corner: Understanding Neuroplasticity

Neuroplasticity is your brain's built-in adaptability. **Focused affirmations**, **mindful movement**, and **consistent practice** can rewire neural pathways, allowing you to replace destructive habits with empowering ones. Research has demonstrated how mindfulness and cognitive training can **strengthen the prefrontal cortex** (the self-control hub) while **reducing reactivity** in the amygdala (the stress center), making it easier to resist cravings,

7

manage emotions, and sustain long term recovery (Tang & Posner, 2015).

The Momhak Method sprang from this insight as a **science-based, self-empowering** approach to real transformation. Traditional recovery has helped millions, but many people seek an alternative path, one that blends cutting-edge research with time-tested practices.

The Momhak 365 Challenge: Transform as You Read

This book encourages **action**, not merely passive page turning. Throughout these chapters, you'll find exercises, reflections, and quick activities designed to help you apply what you're learning in real time.

If you like following a step-by-step plan, turn to **The Momhak 365 Challenge** in Appendix B, which organizes these exercises into a 30-day plan. You can do each exercise as it appears in the chapter, then check off your progress in the Appendix. This way, you never lose momentum—and you *always* have a roadmap for what's next.

First Action Step: Create Your Personal Power Affirmation

Your thoughts shape your reality, so let's build a foundation. You'll use a **Personal Power Affirmation** as a mental anchor—your quick go-to for motivation, focus, or a reset. Let's take a look at how to create yours. It should be:

Positive: Focus on what you want, not what you're avoiding.

Present-Tense: "I *am* strong," rather than "I *will be* strong."

Personal: It should resonate with your unique goals.

Examples:

- "I am strong, clear-headed, and in control."

- "I am calm and focused thriving in sobriety."
- "Every day, I am creating a life I love."

Write it down, say it aloud, or place it somewhere visible. And remember: Your affirmations aren't set in stone. They should evolve alongside your growth and changing needs. What empowers you today may transform as *you* transform, so revisit and refresh your personal power statements as your journey unfolds.

Quick Roadmap for The Momhak Method

This book isn't just about quitting—it's about **rewiring** your brain and **redesigning** your life. Each chapter builds on the last, combining ancient wisdom with modern neuroscience for a step-by-step transformation.

Phase 1: Understanding & Resetting Your Brain

Chapters 1, 2 & 3: Lay the foundation by understanding how addiction affects the brain and taking immediate action through the Four Pillars of The Momhak Method: Moving Meditation, Mind Hacking, Mindful Breathing and Cold Exposure.

Phase 2: Physical & Mental Reset

Chapters 4, 5 & 6: Use powerful physiological and psychological tools—like cold therapy, breathwork, movement and belief reprogramming—to rebuild emotional balance and resilience.

Phase 3: Consistency, Confidence & Connection

Chapters 7 & 8: Strengthen your habits and identity. Learn how to handle real-life triggers, navigate social situations and build routines that reinforce your transformation.

Phase 4: Purpose, Meaning & Long-Term Transformation

Chapters 9 & 10: Move beyond mere sobriety. Rediscover your values, unlock your purpose and design a future aligned with your most powerful, fulfilled self.

How to Use this Book

This isn't a book you'll read once and then shelve. Think of it as your **companion** on the journey to freedom. Here's how to make the most of it:

1. **Follow the Chapters in Order:** Each one builds on the last, giving you a logical path from understanding the problem to fully embracing a new life.

2. **Engage with Exercises: Quick Wins, Momhak Moments**, and guided reflections help you move from insight to action. Keep a notebook or journal handy to record your discoveries.

3. **Explore the Science Corners:** These brief sections illuminate key research or practical tips without overwhelming you. They're your road signs—use them to deepen your knowledge and stay motivated.

4. **Stay Curious:** Approach each section with an open mind. Experiment with the techniques, and don't be afraid to revisit sections if you need a refresher.

Remember: You're the expert of your own experience. The tools and exercises in this book are meant to empower you to steer your recovery—and your life—on *your* terms.

Quick Win: Why Are You Here?

Take 30 seconds right now and ask yourself: ***What brought me to this book today?*** Jot down your top reason. No judgment. This simple reflection can become your bedrock for meaningful change.

Momhak Moment

Sometimes the hardest choice isn't between right or wrong—it's letting go of the old and stepping into the new.

Myth vs. Reality: The Truth About Lasting Change

Myth: "You just need more willpower."
Reality: **Willpower alone often fails when addiction has rewired the brain**. Targeted interventions—like mindful movement or affirmations—can restore balance.

Myth: "Sobriety means giving up a good life."
Reality: **Genuine sobriety isn't about sacrifice**; it's about building a life so fulfilling and balanced that addictive habits lose their hold.

Myth: "If you relapsed before, you'll fail again."
Reality: **Relapse doesn't define your future success**. By addressing both emotional and physical triggers, you can forge a sustainable path forward.

How The Book Is Structured

Each chapter weaves together the informative and incredibly beneficial concepts of:
Understanding Your Brain: Why addiction short-circuits neural pathways, and why pure willpower isn't enough.
Mastering the Physical Reset: Cold exposure, breathwork, and movement to naturally boost dopamine and stabilize mood.
Rewiring the Mind: Science-backed techniques—like affirmations and cognitive reframing—to break negative loops.
Building Your New Life: Routines, habits, and connections that support a healthier, happier you.

In each section, you'll find:

- Personal stories & real-world examples

- **Science Corners** that break things down into plain language

- **Quick Wins** & **Momhak Moments** for motivation

- Step-by-step exercises & reflection prompts

- Practical tips for long-term success

Following this journey will give you not only freedom from addiction but also a comprehensive toolkit for designing a vibrant, purpose-driven life—one in which substances no longer hold any power over you.

"Amazingly, as soon as I stopped drinking and drugging, I became a successful actor. Hollywood called. The rest is history."
—Samuel L. Jackson

Your Journey Starts Here

The road ahead won't be easy; **true change rarely is**. But it'll be worth it. These practices saved my life when nothing else worked, giving me the tools not just to survive but to truly **thrive**. Whether you seek freedom from alcohol, wrestle with other addictive behaviors, or simply crave a new chapter in your life, this book is your roadmap to lasting transformation.

Reminder: Every journey worth taking demands both courage and curiosity. Stay open to new possibilities and embracing new practices, even if they feel uncomfortable at first.

Vision Exercise: Mapping Your Critical Crossroads

Before you dive into Chapter 1, spend 15 to 20 minutes envisioning **two possible futures**—one shaped by inaction, and one driven by the potential within you. I first discovered this exercise in the book *The 30-Day Sobriety Solution,* and it left a lasting impact on me (Andrews & Canfield, 2016).

Find a Quiet Spot: Have a journal or device handy.

Center Yourself: Take three slow breaths: Inhale deeply for four counts, then exhale slowly for six counts.

Embrace Honesty: This is about clarity, not blame or shame.

Part 1: The Path of Continued Struggle

1. Envision Yourself 5 Months from Now If Nothing Changes

- How might your health worsen?

- Which relationships could deteriorate or end?

- How might finances, career, or daily mood suffer?

2. Envision Yourself 5 Years from Now If Nothing Changes

- Any irreversible damage to your health?

- Which dreams or opportunities might be lost?

- Does it echo my brother's fate?

These questions aren't to scare you but instead to highlight where you could find yourself if you remain stuck.

Part 2: The Path of Transformation

1. Envision Yourself 5 Months from Now Embracing The Momhak Method

- How could your energy, sleep, and overall health improve?

- Which habits or skills might make you proud?

- How does each morning feel when you wake up?

- Which friendships or family relationships start to heal or grow stronger?

2. Envision Yourself 5 Years from Now Embracing The Momhak Method

- How might your mind and body flourish?

- Which achievements excite you most?

- How do your closest relationships evolve?

- Which passions have you rekindled or newly discovered?

- How might your financial situation have improved, providing greater security and freedom?

- How does it feel to be fully **alive** in your own life?

Let **hope** and **possibility** guide your pen.

Bridging Vision & Reality
Your Future Starts Now—One Small Step
Change may feel daunting, but you don't need to map your entire future today. Just **take one small step**:

1. Choose One Vision Anchor
Pick one detail from the future you want—just one thing that excites you. Maybe it's waking up clear-headed, reconnecting with an old passion, or feeling physically strong. Write it down and place it where you'll see it daily (on your phone, a sticky note, or your mirror).

2. Take One Immediate Action

- A deep breath before reacting to stress

- A glass of water first thing in the morning

- A two-minute walk outside

- One positive affirmation about yourself

No pressure, no perfection—just movement.

3. Share Your Commitment
You don't have to do this alone. Tell one trusted person about your goal. Or, if you prefer, write it down for yourself. If you feel ready, share your first small win on your socials with **#Momhak365**—because every step forward counts.

Daily Commitment

Whenever you feel old patterns tugging, recall these **two futures**, and ask yourself: *Which future am I choosing right now?*

This isn't just a book—it's a **decision point**. Every page, every exercise, is a step forward.

No more waiting. No more "tomorrow." You've already begun.

Say It Out Loud: "I'm ready to rewire my mind, reset my body, and reclaim my life."

Now, **act**:

- Whisper your intention.

- Try a 10-second cold burst in your next shower.

- Join the **#Momhak365 Challenge**—connect with others who are also rewriting their stories.

CHAPTER 1: THE MOMENT EVERYTHING CHANGED

WHAT YOU'LL DISCOVER

- How a single defining moment can shift your entire path
- Why "rock bottom" is both a wake-up call and a dangerous myth
- The difference between guilt and shame—and how to move forward
- How addiction rewires the brain and why willpower alone won't fix it
- Your decision point: to stay in the cycle or break free

KEY INSIGHTS

- Your brain isn't broken—it's just following an outdated program
- Recognizing your own "moment of truth" is crucial for lasting change
- Addiction isn't a moral failing; it's a **rewiring** of the brain's reward system
- Breathwork and mindfulness can serve as immediate tools for clarity

YOUR TRANSFORMATION TOOLS

- The "**Moment of Truth**" Reflection
- Breathwork for Emotional Reset
- Small First-Step Commitment

"It is not death that a man should fear, but he should fear never beginning to live."
—Marcus Aurelius

A Quiet End

For many of us, real transformation starts with an instant so stark and painful that it can't be ignored. For me, that moment arrived on a deceptively ordinary morning, the day I watched my brother, Casey, take his final breath.

I never imagined that the end would come so quietly. No chaos, no sirens—just a heavy, suffocating calm settling over the space where life used to be, irrevocably separating how things were from how they could never be again.

A Silent Room, A Final Choice

On the day of Casey's death, I showed up at his apartment around 8 a.m., expecting to take him to the hospital for a routine draining of the fluid that was bloating his abdomen. Instead, I walked into his bedroom and found him lying on the bed, covered in blood. The fragile veins in his esophagus—dangerously swollen with blood that was forced to bypass his heavily scarred liver—had ruptured again.

Panic surged. I tried to wrestle him into a wheelchair, to get him to the hospital, but he had no strength. Even more than that, though, he had no inclination to go. When I offered to call an ambulance, he refused. He looked at me, his eyes startlingly clear amidst the wreckage of his body, and simply said, "No." He preferred to stay, to die, rather than continue living the hollowed-out existence that alcohol had left him with.

Seeing his suffering over the last few months—the stick-thin body dominated by a grotesquely swollen stomach, the skeletal face and hollow cheeks, the constant pain, the inability to move or eat—a cold wave of understanding washed over me. His quality of life was gone.

In those harrowing moments, two instincts tore at me: the fierce, primal urge to save him, and the reluctant weight of a promise I'd made weeks earlier. A promise whispered in desperation that if it truly came to this, I'd help him die.

So when I said, "Casey, I should really call an ambulance," he met my gaze, his voice raspy but firm. "Last week," he reminded me, the words hanging heavy in the air, "you were willing to help me die."

I sighed heavily, thick with regret and sadness, realizing that the moment he was resigned to—the moment I'd feared—was now upon us. There was no questioning if it was too late; we both knew that it already was. I clearly remember his bright blue eyes pleading with me to let him die.

And so I did.

I sat with him that morning for hours, just as we had countless times before. Him bleeding, getting weaker and weaker, his breathing getting shallower and shallower. Me drinking a beer and reading Shogun aloud, one of our favorite books, as he bled to death beside me. Periodically, I wiped away the blood he weakly puked up and held his hand, its frailness a stark contrast from the strength I remembered from our countless hours throwing a frisbee or football around.

He finally stopped breathing around 11 that morning. The quietness deepened, becoming absolute. I waited, numb, for almost an hour before calling anyone, wanting to be certain that he couldn't be revived, double-checking for a pulse that wasn't there, just as I'd promised I would. Casey was 46 years old.

Silence. Casey was gone. And I was still here.

If you're feeling overwhelmed reading this, or by anything in your *own* life right now—take a moment with me. Inhale for four counts. Exhale for six. Repeat. That simple act, grounding yourself in your breath, is a reminder: You're here, you're alive, and you always have a choice in how you move forward.

A Wake-Up Call

Casey's death was a brutal awakening I couldn't ignore. Only later, looking back, did I fully grasp what addiction research confirms— that these devastating "rock bottom" moments **can** be catalysts for change; it's just that their power lies not just in the crisis itself but in pairing that raw awakening with concrete steps and unwavering support. Not everyone hits a single, dramatic low; sometimes it's a creeping accumulation of smaller red flags. Either way, transformation often begins only when the current reality becomes truly unbearable.

I'm grateful Casey wasn't alone in his final hours. But he also wasn't alone in how he died. His story is one thread in a vast, tragic tapestry. Nearly 3 million people worldwide die from alcohol-related causes each year (WHO, 2018). In the United States alone, alcohol is responsible for approximately 95,000 deaths annually, making it the third-leading preventable cause of death (NIAAA, 2022).

Behind each number is a name, a face, a family shattered. For many—like Casey—these tragedies might've been prevented with the right information and the right tools, at the right time. Finding those became my mission.

In the immediate aftermath, guilt was a constant shadow. Why hadn't I pushed harder? Could different words, a different action, have saved him? Eventually, I recognized the corrosive difference between guilt and shame. Guilt said, "I could've done more." Shame whispered, "I'm not enough. I'm pathetic." Guilt can motivate change, but shame keeps you trapped. A voice inside reminded me, starkly, that we'd both been floating on the same tidal wave of alcohol dependence, unable to rescue each other because neither of us could fully save ourselves—yet.

Understanding the insidious nature of his illness had brought a painful clarity. In hindsight, the warning signs of end-stage alcoholism had been there, subtle whispers before the final roar. Extra fatigue he'd brushed off, occasional stomach aches numbed by another beer… these were the faint signals of alcohol-related liver disease creeping in. By the time the symptoms screamed crisis, irreversible damage had been done.

Understanding End-Stage Alcoholism

His first close call had come years earlier, around his 40th birthday. Feeling unwell, he'd reached for his usual remedy—beer—only to start vomiting massive amounts of blood. At the hospital, doctors found a ruptured vein in his throat ("esophageal varices" in medical terms). His liver was already so scarred that blood, unable to flow through it properly, was backing up, engorging these fragile veins. The first visible sign had been a black, tar-like stool days earlier—a classic indicator of internal bleeding. (If you ever see this in your own stool, seek medical help immediately.)

Over the following years, his condition deteriorated despite interventions. The scarred liver couldn't process fluids, causing ascites—severe abdominal bloating requiring painful, monthly draining. The blood continued to bypass the liver, swelling those esophageal veins like ticking time bombs. When they burst, it was catastrophic.

What made Casey's story particularly striking, even to me, was how he defied the common "alcoholic" stereotype. Outwardly, he seemed relatively fit. We'd spend afternoons throwing a ball around and take long walks around his Vancouver neighborhood. He rarely got visibly, falling-down drunk, and his drink of choice was beer, not hard liquor. But in a culture that often normalizes and even glamorizes certain kinds of drinking—craft beer festivals, wine pairings, weekend binges—his story is a harsh reminder that slow, steady intake can inflict devastating internal damage, masked by a facade of normalcy until it's far too late.

The Path That Led Us Here

His winding road, in many ways, mirrored my own. We grew up in an environment where heavy drinking wasn't just normal; it was often celebrated. We both wrestled with alcohol, both tried—and failed at—moderation countless times. I'd manage weeks, sometimes months of abstinence, only to slide back into the same destructive pattern: typically a 15-pack of beer a day, but often more.

Every day that you delay addressing a pattern like this, you reinforce the old neural pathways, making them more deeply entrenched. Addiction doesn't just fade away; it actively hijacks the brain's reward and control systems. The longer you wait, the harder it feels to break free. But here's the crucial truth: The instant you decide to act, *everything* begins to shift. Even the smallest step—admitting a difficult truth, choosing water over wine tonight, or finally making that call—can set a radically different future in motion.

If you've struggled with moderation, you understand the cycle of hope and frustration. You know how baffling it is when willpower inevitably fails against the relentless pull of dependence. Let's explore **why** that approach so often falls short for those truly caught in alcohol's grip.

Momhak Moment

Understanding the science doesn't erase the pain, but it shows a way through it. Knowledge becomes power the moment we use it.

Science Corner: Understanding Moderation Attempts

Heavy drinking rewires your brain. Over time, alcohol creates strong habit loops that link stress, cravings, and reward. According to Seo and Sinha (2015), this makes moderation extremely hard—your brain starts to want more, not less, even when you try to cut back.

Moderation is the tempting middle ground: we want to hold onto the parts of drinking that feel pleasurable—bonding with friends, taking the edge off stress—while sidestepping the negative consequences. But when alcohol becomes wired into your brain's sense of reward, the "just one drink" mantra can trigger a cascade of cravings that's nearly impossible to shut down.

I'd fallen for that trap more times than I could count. I'd tried cutting back, placing arbitrary limits, swearing off hard liquor while still drinking beer—each time convincing myself I could control it. And each time, I ended up right back where I'd started.

Sobriety Is Strength: Proof from the World's Most Successful People

Sobriety isn't a limitation—it's a gateway to strength, clarity, and success. Many of the world's most accomplished individuals have chosen to live alcohol and drug-free lives. Their stories prove that giving up substances isn't about sacrifice—it's about stepping into your fullest potential. Below are some examples of successful sober individuals who've built extraordinary lives without relying on substances.

Actors & Entertainers

- **Robert Downey Jr.** – After years of substance abuse, Downey Jr. has been sober since 2003, crediting martial arts and family support for helping him reclaim his life and career.

- **Samuel L. Jackson** – Jackson has been sober since 1991, turning his life around after a drug overdose and going on to become one of the highest-grossing actors of all time.

- **Brad Pitt** – Pitt has been sober since 2016, sharing that quitting alcohol allowed him to reconnect with himself and his family.

- **Gerard Butler** – Butler has spoken about how quitting alcohol over two decades ago allowed him to build a successful acting career and improve his mental health.

- **Ewan McGregor** – McGregor has been sober since 2001, citing that quitting alcohol helped him focus on his career and personal relationships.

- **Jim Carrey** – Carrey quit alcohol and drugs years ago, explaining that sobriety allowed him to reconnect with his creativity and emotional balance.

- **Colin Farrell** – Farrell has been sober since 2006, crediting his recovery for helping him manage depression and build a stable life.

- **Tobey Maguire** – The actor has been sober since the early 2000s, explaining that sobriety helped him maintain balance and success.

- **Bradley Cooper** – Cooper gave up drinking in 2004, calling it the foundation for his professional and personal growth.

- **Anne Hathaway** – Hathaway quit alcohol in 2019, explaining that alcohol didn't serve her life or her goals anymore.

- **Alec Baldwin** – Baldwin has been sober since 1985, crediting Alcoholics Anonymous for helping him regain control over his life.

- **John Goodman** – Goodman gave up alcohol in 2007, sharing that giving up alcohol saved both his health and his career.

- **James Franco** – Franco has been sober since the early 2000s, turning to art and writing as creative outlets for healing.

Musicians

- **Eminem** – The rapper has been sober since 2008 after nearly dying from an overdose, and he's credited his sobriety for saving his life and inspiring his music.

- **Eric Clapton** – Clapton hasn't touched alcohol since 1987, and he even founded a rehabilitation center to help others recover from addiction.

- **Elton John** – Elton has been sober since 1990 and frequently shares how his recovery transformed his life and career.

- **Adele** – Adele quit drinking in 2019, explaining that sobriety improved her emotional stability and creativity.

- **Jessica Simpson** – Simpson has been sober since 2017, explaining that giving up alcohol allowed her to reclaim her life and confidence.

- **50 Cent** – The rapper has stated that he avoids alcohol and drugs entirely, focusing on fitness and business instead.

- **Naomi Campbell** – Campbell quit drinking after years of struggling with addiction, crediting her sobriety for stabilizing her mental health.

- **Stephen King** – King has been sober since 1987, sharing that quitting drugs and alcohol saved both his life and his writing career.

- **Eva Mendes** – Mendes entered recovery in 2008 and has been sober ever since, explaining that sobriety allowed her to refocus on her career and family.

Athletes

- **Terry Crews** – Crews has been sober from alcohol, as well as pornography, since 2009, calling sobriety a crucial part of his personal and professional success.

- **Steve Austin** – The professional wrestler quit drinking and has credited sobriety with improving his health and mental clarity.

- **Dennis Rodman** – Rodman has notoriously struggled with addiction in the past but has been sober since undergoing treatment in recent years.

- **Andy Murray** – The tennis champion has maintained a sober lifestyle, crediting his disciplined approach to training and mental health.

Comedians & Public Figures

- **Dane Cook** – Cook has been sober for over two decades, explaining that alcohol didn't align with his goals or lifestyle.

- **Tyra Banks** – Banks has never consumed alcohol or drugs, saying that staying clear-headed was important to her success.

- **Blake Lively** – Lively also says that she's never touched alcohol or drugs, explaining that sobriety aligns with her natural lifestyle and career goals.

- **Megan Fox** – Fox quit drinking after realizing that alcohol was negatively affecting her health and mental clarity.

- **Jada Pinkett Smith** – Pinkett Smith has been sober for years, explaining that sobriety was crucial for her mental and emotional health.

- **Natalie Portman** – Portman has shared that she gave up alcohol after college, explaining that it didn't serve her life.

- **Warren Buffet** – Buffet has maintained a sober lifestyle for most of his life, focusing on discipline and long-term success.

- **Donald Trump** – Trump has openly stated that he's never consumed alcohol, citing his older brother's struggles with alcoholism as a reason for his choice.

- **Craig Ferguson** – Sober since 1992, Ferguson openly discusses his alcoholism, stating that he's one of the "certain types of people [who] can't drink" and requires ongoing effort to manage his recovery.

These individuals didn't give up substances to limit themselves; they made the choice to thrive. Their success stories prove that sobriety is often the key to unlocking personal growth, creative excellence, and long-term success.

The decision to quit drinking or using substances isn't about weakness—it's about strength and empowerment. If these high achievers can find success and clarity in sobriety, so can you.

The Moment Everything Shifted

But even knowing that others have found strength in sobriety, the decision to quit can feel deeply personal and uncertain. For me, the turning point wasn't just about giving up alcohol—it was about finding a new way to engage with life.

That's when I started experimenting with something different. Instead of relying on willpower alone, I discovered how to work with my brain's natural ability to change—or what scientists call "neuroplasticity." Think of your brain as a series of well-worn hiking trails. Each time you act on a habit—good or bad—you tread that path more deeply, making it easier to follow next time. Recovery is akin to forging new trails in a dense forest. It takes time, consistency, and the willingness to walk unfamiliar routes. But once these healthier neural pathways are established, they become your new default.

Science Corner: The Neuroscience of Transformation

Though addiction alters brain circuits, these same circuits can be **rewired** through comprehensive interventions that combine behavioral, physical, and psychological methods. Tools like affirmations, cold exposure, breathwork, and mindful movement form **new neural pathways** that gradually replace old defaults. This principle forms the foundation of The Momhak Method— **building new, life-affirming habits** to reshape both mind and behavior.

Momhak Moment

Sobriety doesn't take away your edge—it sharpens it.

Guilt, Regret & Moving Forward

Casey's death shattered me, but it also revealed a truth I couldn't ignore: *If I didn't change, I was next.* The past was unchangeable, but my future was still mine to shape.

I'd wanted to save Casey, but at that time, I couldn't even save myself. In the wake of his death, something had shifted. I realized I had a choice: I could continue spiraling down the same path, or I could break the cycle. I chose the latter.

Right now, **you** stand at a similar crossroads. One road takes you back to the pain, the regret, and the chaos. The other leads to clear-headed mornings, empowerment, and freedom.

Choosing a different path can feel daunting, and almost isolating at first. But you need to know that countless others are taking this step right now as well, sharing their own Day 1 commitment or their first small win by using **#Momhak365**.

The Biology of Rock Bottom

Hitting rock bottom may be necessary for some, but it's also incredibly dangerous. Addiction hijacks your brain's ability to see the truth. The deeper you go, the harder it gets to recognize the way out—but neuroplasticity proves that you can rewire your mind for freedom. And I saw this paradox play out firsthand in my own life.

"Rock bottom became the solid foundation on which I rebuilt my life."
—J.K. Rowling

My Own Rock Bottom

Over the years, my relationship with alcohol had cost me—*dearly*. I crashed a car, got divorced, and sold a house I loved (mostly to cover debts). My mental health drastically declined. Physical detox became so brutal that I'd shake uncontrollably, unable to feed myself during the worst of it—and even if I could, food wouldn't stay down. Hallucinations of giant insects crawling on the walls twisted my perception, making it nearly impossible to discern reality.

At one point, I went to the hospital "just to ask about detox options," and they immediately checked me in, seeing how close I was to disaster. Each time I tried to quit using sheer willpower, I'd eventually convince myself I could handle "just one drink," only to find myself back at the bottom in just a few short days, drinking a 15-pack a day with the usual vodka-Jager chasers.

Science Corner: Understanding Withdrawal

Chronic alcohol use disrupts the brain's delicate balance of neurotransmitters, especially GABA (calming) and glutamate (stimulating). As Koob and Volkow (2016) explain in *The Lancet Psychiatry*, this disruption creates a volatile rebound effect during withdrawal—raising the risk of tremors, hallucinations, and even seizures. If you're physically dependent on alcohol, don't go it alone: Seek medical guidance before quitting cold turkey.

The Turning Point

Looking back at my brother's death stirs complex emotions. While the grief and regret run deep, that devastating moment gave me a piercing clarity I'd never experienced. There at his cremation, sharing a final drink with our surviving brother, I faced an unavoidable truth: I could continue down Casey's path, or I could choose life. In that moment of both tribute and finality, I raised my glass one last time—not just to honor Casey's memory, but to mark the end of my own relationship with alcohol.

That final drink was a symbolic turning point. On one hand, it was a toast to the closeness we'd once shared; on the other, it was a stark farewell to the substance that had stolen so much from both of us. Walking away from that moment felt like stepping out of a burning building, fully aware of the heat still licking at my back but resolute *never* to go back in. The sense of finality I felt that day was fueled by emotion, but the next step—rewiring my brain—was grounded in science.

Momhak Moment

Our darkest hours can be our greatest teachers if we choose to learn from them. Pain alone doesn't cause growth, but it often cracks the door where transformation becomes possible.

In the chapters ahead, you'll see how I transitioned from that grim scene to a life rich in mindful, healthy habits. I combined ancient wisdom—yoga, Chi Gong, meditation—with modern neuroscience like affirmations, cold exposure, and breathwork. These tools didn't just keep me sober; they built a life so fulfilling that I no longer felt the urge to escape.

Could I have saved Casey? I'll never know. But I *can* save myself— and perhaps by sharing my story and method, I can help you, too.

Your Journey Forward

Many people try to overcome addiction by simply **eliminating** the substance, assuming that willpower is enough. Too often though, it isn't. Real transformation demands a **total recalibration** of mind, body, and spirit. If you're reading this, you've likely sensed that "just quitting" or attending a few meetings won't get you to the life you want.

Stopping is critical, but **healing** the root wounds is what deters relapse. That involves compassion for yourself, understanding your brain's wiring, and crafting habits aligned with your deepest values.

"When everything seems to be going against you, remember that the airplane takes off against the wind, not with it."
—Henry Ford

For a step-by-step framework on incorporating these ideas into daily life, see the **Momhak 365 Challenge** in the Appendix.

A Look at the Methods I Tried

Early on, I explored several standard recovery methods, each with pros but none that fully matched my needs:

Willpower Alone

I initially relied solely on willpower, believing that sheer determination would suffice. While willpower is essential, addiction often rewires the brain's reward system, making it challenging to resist cravings through mere determination. This approach led to repeated relapses, highlighting the need for a more comprehensive strategy.

The Sinclair Method

This technique involves taking a particular medication to reduce the pleasurable effects of alcohol. Despite its success for some, it didn't yield the desired results for me. The method's focus on pharmacological intervention didn't address the underlying psychological and emotional aspects of my addiction.

Alcoholics Anonymous (AA)

AA is a lifeline for many, but I found it challenging for several reasons:

- **Pandemic Restrictions:** The COVID-19 pandemic limited in-person meetings, but even before this restriction, the meetings just didn't resonate with me.

- **Introversion:** As an introvert, sharing personal experiences in group settings was daunting, making it difficult to fully engage.

- **Spiritual Emphasis:** The program's emphasis on a higher power was a barrier for me and others I know—including my brother, who felt uncomfortable with the spiritual undertones.

- **The Powerlessness Concept:** I struggled with AA's first step of admitting powerlessness over addiction. I believe that while addiction is incredibly difficult to overcome, true recovery comes from recognizing your own inner strength and capacity for change. You aren't powerless—you simply need effective tools and understanding to harness your inherent ability to transform. The methods I describe in this book empower you to recognize both the challenge and your capability to overcome it.

Realizing that no single, uniform approach would work for me, I created The Momhak Method—**Mind Hacking, Cold Exposure, Mindful Breathing, and Moving Meditation**—crafted to resonate with my personality. It led me to a sustainable, **freedom-based** sobriety.

The Momhak Method: A Sneak Peek

- **Mind Hacking**: Rewiring your mental patterns through powerful thought-reframing techniques and strategic affirmations that transform your subconscious programming.

- **Mindful Breathing**: Techniques for stress relief, cravings, and anxiety control.

- **Moving Meditation**: Yoga, Tai Chi, or mindful walks, syncing breath and motion for holistic well-being.

- **Cold Exposure**: Gradual, safe methods to tap into your body's resilience, resetting dopamine levels.

It's not about white-knuckling sobriety; it's about **building** a life worth staying sober for—full of excitement and growth. At any point, you can decide to change. Casey's story shows how fleeting life can be—but mine shows how quickly it can be reclaimed. If you're even just slightly on the fence, let that uncertainty open you to discovery. Keep turning these pages, and let's walk this path **together**, one hopeful step at a time.

Chapter 1 Summary: The Moment Everything Changed

Core Message

Transformation begins with a stark moment of truth, but *true* change unfolds when you act on that realization.

Key Lessons

Your brain isn't broken: Addiction is a rewiring, not a moral failing.

Rock bottom isn't mandatory—*clarity* is: A crisis can spark action, but awareness alone can be enough.

Pain can be a teacher or a prison: The hardest moments can trap us or propel us toward transformation.

Your #Momhak365 Challenge: Choose Your Path

Right now, you stand at a crossroads.

One path loops back to where you've been, but **another** can start right now.

Before you do anything else:

1. Write down one hard truth about your habit.

2. Take just one single step today: A deep breath, texting a friend, or journaling for 5 minutes.

You don't need to know everything yet—just decide which **future** you're aiming for.

Bonus: Share your first step using **#Momhak365**. Public commitments can amplify progress.

Mindful Moment: A Decision in Your Body

1. Close your eyes. Inhale for 4 seconds, exhale for 6.

2. Visualize yourself 5 years from now if nothing changes. How does that feel?

3. Now imagine 5 years from now if you embrace this path. What's different?

4. Realize that your choices today shape tomorrow's reality.

Embody Your Choice: Stand up. Take one deep 4–6 breath. As you exhale, consciously **choose** your path of transformation. You might gently clench your fist in resolve, place a hand over your heart, or simply stand taller. Hold that physical intention for 5 seconds. Acknowledge this decision **in your body** before sitting back down.

It may seem overwhelming, but you don't need to overhaul your life overnight. The next chapters break everything into **manageable** steps, showing you how addiction hijacks your brain—and how you can take it back without relying on raw willpower alone.

Looking Ahead: The Truth About Willpower

A lot of people pause here at this point, believing that they just need to try harder. Chapter 2 exposes why that mindset generally fails—and how you can **reset** your brain for genuine change:

- **Why** can quitting feel impossible even when you want it?

- **How** does addiction hijack your reward system?

- **Which** science-backed tools help you break free?

Cravings don't control you—your brain is waiting for new instructions.

CHAPTER 2: THE SCIENCE OF ADDICTION & CHANGE

WHAT YOU'LL DISCOVER

- Why willpower alone keeps failing you (and what really works)
- How addiction hijacks your brain's reward system
- The science of neuroplasticity—your brain's natural reset button
- Practical tools to rewire cravings and build new neural pathways

KEY INSIGHTS

- Your brain isn't broken—it's just running outdated programming
- Addiction is about dopamine, not moral failure
- You can rebuild your pleasure response naturally

YOUR TRANSFORMATION TOOLS

- The **Dopamine Audit** exercise
- Science-backed affirmations that actually work
- Quick-win strategies for immediate relief
- Practical exercises to strengthen your recovery

"Neurons that fire together wire together."
—Donald Hebb, neuropsychologist and neuroplasticity pioneer

Beyond Willpower

You wake up telling yourself, *Today's the day. No more drinking*. The morning feels fresh with possibility. But by noon, you feel an itch crawling under your skin. By nightfall, that old familiar thought sneaks in: *Just one*. Before you know it, you're pouring a drink. Then two. Then three… until your resolve crumbles completely and the familiar bargaining begins: *Well, if this is my last night drinking, I might as well go all out*. The next morning arrives with a vengeance—your head pounding, your stomach churning, and that crushing weight of regret pressing down on your chest yet again.

Why does this happen, even when you're desperate for change? Modern neuroscience reveals a pivotal truth: It's not about willpower; it's about how addiction hijacks your brain's reward circuits. The good news? You can **rewire** those circuits using techniques that blend ancient wisdom and cutting-edge science.

Quick Win: Understanding Your Brain

Take a moment to recall the last time you tried to quit or moderate a habit.

What triggered your relapse? (Stress? Social event? Boredom?)

How did you feel in the moment it happened?

Write down a few notes. Recognizing triggers is your **first step** toward reprogramming them.

Extra Insight: Also, note how you felt afterward (disappointment, shame, resignation, etc.). These emotional responses can perpetuate the cycle.

The Hidden Truth About Addiction

For years, I saw my inability to stop drinking as a **personal weakness**. Maybe you've felt it, too—the shame of wondering why you can't just quit when others can. But neuroscience tells a more empowering story: Addiction isn't a moral failing; it's an **overactive**

reward system doing what it evolved to do—just at an intensity that nature never intended.

Momhak Moment

Remember: Your brain isn't broken—it's just following outdated instructions. But the good news is that you can rewrite the code. **Why This Matters**: Understanding your brain's adaptation to substance use can replace shame with curiosity. Instead of blaming yourself, you're motivated to tackle the root cause—your neural wiring.

The Dopamine Story: Your Brain's Secret Controller

Your brain isn't addicted to alcohol itself—it's addicted to the **massive dopamine rush** that alcohol unleashes. Here's the cycle, broken down and simplified:

1. **Alcohol equals a dopamine explosion.** Your brain experiences an unnatural high.

2. **Your brain fights back.** It lowers dopamine receptor levels, making everyday pleasures feel dull.

3. **You drink more.** Not necessarily because you crave it, but to feel "normal" again.

This is why quitting feels so miserable early on—your brain needs time to **heal** and relearn how to enjoy everyday rewards, like sunshine or a satisfying meal.

When I first discovered that cravings weren't just "bad habits" but actual neural pathways lighting up my brain's reward circuit, I felt both relieved and frustrated. Relieved, because I realized I wasn't just "weak," but frustrated because I had to accept that my brain chemistry was working against me—*unless* I learned how to reset it. This moment changed my perspective on willpower forever.

Emotional Triggers Behind Cravings

Cravings aren't purely chemical—they're also about **emotional coping**. If it were only about neurochemistry, just waiting out withdrawal might do the trick. But the truth is, **many of us drink, smoke, or use substances not just for the high but also to numb something deeper**. These emotions include:

- **Stress** – Unwinding after a hard day

- **Anxiety** – Taking the edge off social situations

- **Depression** – Trying to escape sadness or numbness

- **Loneliness** – Filling empty moments with substance use

- **Boredom** – Passing time without meaningful engagement

When these root emotions remain unaddressed, they fuel cravings. The brain recalls the temporary relief, and so the minute when discomfort surfaces, it nudges you back to the old escape route. **Remember:** True freedom demands addressing the underlying emotional pain, not merely discarding the substance.

Chronic Use, Lower Baseline Dopamine

Research in *The New England Journal of Medicine* shows that long-term substance use reshapes the brain's dopamine system, lowering natural pleasure levels and making it harder to enjoy everyday activities (Volkow et al., 2016)

Reflection Exercise: Mapping Emotional Cravings

Think back to your last craving or relapse. Instead of just focusing on **what** triggered it (e.g., "I was at a party" or "I was stressed"), dig deeper:

Which emotions were you feeling? (Loneliness, boredom, anxiety?)

What did you hope the substance would provide? (Relief, social ease, distraction?)

Could anything else have helped? (Calling a friend, exercising, or journaling?)

Write down your answers. You might start to see a pattern. Identifying the **emotional driver** behind cravings is the key to replacing destructive habits with healthier ones.

The Unwind Ritual That Almost Broke Me

I had a job many people would envy—working outdoors as an archaeologist, uncovering history's secrets under the open sky. But even dream jobs have their stresses: the pressure of deadlines, the physical demands, the detailed record keeping. By the time I'd get home, my body was exhausted from the fieldwork and my mind was full of unfinished tasks. Every cell seemed to cry out for relief. "Just a few drinks to take the edge off," I'd whisper to myself. It was a lie I'd perfected.

That first sip felt like magic—cold, soothing, and hitting a reset button in my overwhelmed brain. The second drink melted away the day's tension, but something else disappeared, too—my clarity and my control. By drink six, my problems seemed distant and blurry. By drink eight, I couldn't care less about tomorrow's consequences.

I told myself I was being responsible. This wasn't about getting drunk – this was "stress management," my reward for surviving another day. I had it under control. Until I didn't.

What started as a choice transformed into a ritual, and then the ritual became a requirement. And stress? That was just my favorite excuse.

Soon a terrible pattern emerged: drink to numb today's stress, wake up to find it doubled tomorrow, then drink more to handle the amplified pressure. Round and round it went, each cycle digging me deeper into a hole I couldn't see.

Then came the moment that shattered my illusions. One perfectly normal evening—no stress, no drama, and for no reason at all—I felt that familiar itch crawling under my skin, demanding its daily dose. That's when the truth hit me: *This has nothing to do with stress anymore. My brain's been rewired, programmed to crave alcohol like a computer running on corrupted code.*

Alcohol wasn't my stress reliever—it was my stress multiplier, stealing my peace one evening at a time.

I didn't quit that day, but something had shifted. I began experimenting with alternatives: deep, conscious breathing when anxiety struck; shocking my system with cold water; and taking mindful walks to process my thoughts.

Looking back, I now realize my brain has always been fast-moving, restless, and hard to quiet—what many today would call ADHD. I never had that label growing up, but I see now how much it shaped my choices, especially my turn toward substances that seemed to calm the chaos. If that sounds familiar, you're not alone. For some of us, addiction wasn't about numbing pain or dealing with stress—it was about slowing down a brain that never stops moving.

These simple tools seemed almost laughably basic at first. But here's what I discovered: Unlike alcohol, they actually *worked*. And best of all? They left my mornings intact, giving me back those precious hours alcohol had been stealing for years.

Today, my mind still moves quickly—but it's no longer out of control. Through breathwork, movement, and dopamine resets, I've found a rhythm that works. I feel calmer, more focused, and far less scattered than I ever did before.

Quick Reflection: Your Own Unwind Ritual

Have you ever used alcohol (or another habit) to "unwind"?

Which stressors drive you to that decision?

Does it actually relieve stress, or just **postpone** and **multiply** it?

What's one healthier way to de-stress that won't leave you feeling worse tomorrow?

The Price of Artificial Pleasure

As dopamine receptors "turn down," two major problems emerge:

1. **Escalating Use:** You need more of the substance—more drinks, more often—to achieve the same high.

2. **Diminished Natural Joy:** Activities that once felt rewarding (like hobbies or time with friends) lose their spark.

Everyday Example: Someone who used to love weekend hikes now finds them "not worth the effort." Their reward system is so **hijacked** that normal joys feel flat.

"Originally, I was a happy drunk. But later I was miserable because it's a depressant. I was ashamed of myself, really."
—Ewan McGregor

Science Corner: Your Brain's Built-In Reset Button

Neuroimaging studies confirm that your brain can rewire itself (Volkow et al., 2016). Addiction may carve deep pathways in your reward system, but those patterns aren't permanent. The same brain scans that reveal these changes also show that they can be reversed. With consistent tools—like affirmations, mindful movement, cold exposure, and breathwork—you can build new, healthier circuits.

Try This: The Dopamine Audit

1. For the next 24 hours, note anything that gives you a small jolt of pleasure—maybe coffee, a favorite song, or a text from a friend.

2. Rate it from 1–10.

3. Do the same during a week without alcohol. Notice if your natural pleasures start feeling stronger by the end of the week.

THC, Dopamine & Recovery: A Potential Complication

For many, quitting alcohol or other substances leaves a void, and THC (cannabis) can seem like an appealing alternative, especially with increasing accessibility and social acceptance. Often viewed as a more "natural" or less harmful option than alcohol for managing stress or sleep, it doesn't carry the same risks of severe withdrawal or organ damage.

But this seemingly simpler substitute isn't always straightforward in recovery. While THC provides a temporary dopamine boost and potentially offers short-term relief, it can also complicate the brain's healing process. Over time, relying on it can lower baseline motivation and pleasure, and what starts as an occasional aid might become a daily habit, substituting one dependency for another. In my own experience, while it initially felt less harmful than alcohol, THC became another way to numb emotions rather than process them, slowing down the deeper rewiring my brain needed.

The effects of THC vary greatly from person to person. Is it a helpful bridge, or does it hinder deeper recovery by masking underlying issues? Because this is such a nuanced topic with significant personal variability, we'll explore it in much greater detail a little later in the book. Chapter 8 delves deeper into the complex role of THC in recovery—including its impact on social settings, relapse risks, and potential benefits—and provides a framework to help you assess whether it aligns with your personal recovery goals.

For now, just recognize that like any substance affecting dopamine, its use requires careful consideration.

And remember: Always consult with a medical or mental health professional if you have questions about substance use in your recovery journey.

Exercise: The Clean Dopamine Boost

While substances flood your brain with dopamine—only to leave you depleted and craving more—exercise offers something different. Dr. Anna Lembke, author of *Dopamine Nation* and head of Stanford's Addiction Medicine Clinic, explains that physical activity is one of the few natural behaviors that provides a meaningful dopamine boost without a crash (2021). That's what makes it such a powerful tool for recovery: You get the reward without the withdrawal.

Science Corner: Exercise & Brain Chemistry

Evidence shows that exercise:

- **Regulates** dopamine receptors

- **Reduces** stress hormones like cortisol

- **Supports** overall mental well-being

Crucially, it avoids the **high-low** cycle of substance use, and instead fosters **sustainable** improvements in mood and resilience.

The Exercise Advantage

Substances	vs.	Exercise
spike dopamine **unnaturally high**	vs.	boosts dopamine **naturally**
force the brain to **reduce** dopamine receptors	vs.	maintains **healthy** receptor function

leave you needing **more**	vs.	creates **lasting** mood improvements

Finding Your Movement

The key is finding physical activities that resonate with you personally. For instance, I love hiking, stand-up paddle boarding, and surfing. Activities that might resonate with you include:

- Walking and hiking

- Gardening

- Yoga or stretching

- Swimming or cycling

- Team sports

- Any movement that feels sustainable and enjoyable

The best exercise program is one that you'll actually stick with. Just start where you are and build gradually.

The Impact of Resentment & Forgiveness on Well-Being

Research on emotional well-being and neuroscience suggests that holding onto resentment can have negative physiological and psychological effects. Studies indicate that chronic stress, often fueled by unresolved anger and grudges, can activate the body's stress response, leading to increased cortisol levels, heightened cravings, and diminished impulse control. This, in turn, may contribute to relapse in individuals recovering from addiction. On the other hand, **forgiveness has been associated with various health benefits**, including reduced stress, improved emotional regulation, and better cardiovascular health. Practicing forgiveness—whether toward oneself or others—has been linked to lower blood pressure, decreased anxiety, and enhanced overall well-being. While research continues to explore its full impact on

46

addiction recovery, many experts agree that releasing resentment helps promote mental clarity, resilience, and emotional balance.

The Role of Forgiveness in Emotional & Neural Healing

While the neuroscience of forgiveness is still developing, studies suggest that letting go of deep-seated grudges may help regulate stress responses and improve emotional wellness. Forgiveness can reduce rumination (a key factor in anxiety and depression) and encourage the development of healthier coping mechanisms. Emotional healing through forgiveness doesn't mean excusing harmful behavior—it means freeing yourself from the emotional burdens that reinforce negative cycles.

Forgiveness in addiction recovery is particularly powerful. Many who struggle with substance use also battle feelings of guilt, shame, or regret. In particular, self-forgiveness allows us to move forward without being trapped by past mistakes, which can be a crucial factor in sustaining long-term sobriety.

Remember: Forgiveness isn't about excusing harm—it's about reclaiming personal freedom. Letting go of resentment can ease emotional burdens, reduce stress, and support long-term healing.

Momhak Moment

Holding onto resentment is like swallowing poison and expecting someone else to get sick. The weight of unforgiveness burdens only the one who carries it.

Beyond the Victim Mindset

Dr. Lembke emphasizes the importance of personal responsibility in recovery. Seeing yourself as a helpless victim, she explains, undermines your brain's ability to heal. This philosophy aligns closely with Dr. Carol Dweck's growth mindset research, which shows that viewing challenges as opportunities for growth significantly improves long-term outcomes (2006).

Those who approach adversity as a chance to learn—rather than an unjust burden—generally show:

- Greater resilience to stress

- Higher success in long-term goals

- Better life satisfaction

- Stronger recovery rates

Momhak Moment

Your struggles aren't punishments—they're invitations to grow. Each challenge can become a stepping stone to transformation.

Practical Applications in Recovery

Recognize Your Power: Shift I'm stuck in addiction to *I'm learning new tools to reclaim control.*

View Setbacks as Data: Instead of thinking things like, *I failed again,* ask yourself, *What triggers does this reveal?*

Take Responsibility Without Shame: Acknowledge your role but let go of destructive self-blame.

The Recovery Paradox

The more we accept responsibility for our recovery—while letting go of shame about our past—the more likely we are to succeed. It's about **empowerment**, not blame.

Remember this: Cravings don't mean that you're failing—they mean that your brain is healing.

Next time a craving appears, don't just resist it—**observe** it:

- **What triggered** this urge? (Stress, boredom, social pressure?)

- **What** do I want to feel? (Relief, excitement, numbness?)

- **What happens** if I give in? (Momentary relief, long-term regret?)

- **What happens** if I don't? (Pride, better sleep, more confidence?)

Tracking these patterns grants you power over them.

Affirmations can serve as a shield. The instant you feel the urge, a statement like "I am strong and calm" or "I am relaxed thriving in sobriety" can disrupt the loop, allowing your rational brain to step in.

Breaking the Cycle

Your brain's reward system is powerful, and fighting it with sheer willpower is like trying to stop a flood with your hands. The Momhak Method uses a smarter approach—working with your brain's natural processes, using proven techniques to steadily shift your neural pathways toward healthier patterns.

The Momhak Method Advantage

While traditional recovery often focuses on **what you're giving up**, The Momhak Method emphasizes what you're **gaining**—fresh neural pathways, rejuvenated natural pleasures, and an expanded toolbox for stress.

Empowerment vs. Deprivation: Reframing "I can't drink" into "I get to live fully thriving in sobriety" can lighten the emotional weight of change.

Affirmation Exercise: Rewire Your Inner Voice

Morning: Say your **Personal Power Affirmation** while looking in the mirror (e.g., "I am strong and healthy, thriving in sobriety. My mind is clear, and my body is energized.")

During Stress Trigger: Pair a short affirmation with extended exhale 4–6 breathing (e.g., "I handle challenges calmly and confidently. I have the tools to stay centered.")

The Science of Affirmations

Affirmations aren't just positive thinking—they're actually neuroscience as well. Research from UCLA and Stanford shows that self-affirmation activates reward centers in the brain, boosts motivation, and helps buffer stress. In one Stanford study, students who practiced affirmations daily showed better academic performance and lower stress levels (Cohen & Sherman, 2014). The same principles apply in habit change and addiction recovery: When you affirm who you're becoming, your brain starts to believe it.

Remember to craft powerful affirmations that are believable, present tense ("I am... "), personally meaningful, and expressed with emotion. Repeating them regularly—especially at key times like waking, bedtime, or during stress—helps reshape neural pathways for positive change.

I like to combine affirmations with Tummo/Wim Hof breath holds—it amplifies and deepens the experience.

Tools for Rewiring

Below are the four essential reprogramming strategies:

1. Cold Exposure

- Naturally boosts dopamine

- Builds resilience by exposing you to controlled stress

- Associates "challenge" with "growth"

2. Moving Meditation

- Yoga, Qi Gong, or mindful walking unify body & mind

- Releases endorphins while promoting calm

- Fosters positive connections with mindful activity

3. Mindful Breathing

- Activates your parasympathetic "rest and digest" system

- Boosts prefrontal cortex function (key for decision-making)

- Offers a quick, portable craving-buster

4. Mind Hacking (Affirmations, Cognitive Reframing, Pain-Pleasure Reset)

- Rewires negative self-talk

- Strengthens confidence and motivation circuits

- Elicits emotion, flagging importance to your brain

- Customizes your personal journey

- Integrates breathwork, cold therapy, and journaling

5. Journaling (Honorary 5th Tool)

- Processes emotions and reveals hidden triggers

- Encourages self-reflection, and solidifying insights

- Tracks progress and reinforces commitment

Your Personal Experiment

Reflection Exercise: Understanding Your Patterns
Take 10 minutes to outline your day

Natural Pleasure Moments: Times you genuinely feel good

Trigger Situations: Times or places that nudge you toward a negative habit

Current Coping Mechanisms: How do you handle stress or boredom now?

New Habit Options: Where could you insert a short walk, affirmation, or breathwork?

Expanded Tip: Create short labels for your triggers (e.g., "Evening Stress Trigger" or "Social Anxiety Trigger"). Recognizing them quickly helps you activate an affirmation or breathing exercise before your old habit takes hold.

Putting It All Into Practice

Now that you understand how addiction hijacks your brain—and how **neuroplasticity** offers a route to freedom—you're equipped with new insights. The coming chapters reveal how to integrate these tools into a daily routine that feels both doable and fulfilling.

Chapter 2 Summary: The Science of Addiction & Change

Core Message

Addiction isn't about willpower—it's about how your brain has been rewired. And the good news is that you can reprogram it.

Key Lessons

Your brain is addicted to dopamine, not just substances like alcohol. Substances hijack your reward system, overshadowing everyday joys.

Willpower fails because your brain works against you. Knowing how dopamine and neuroplasticity work opens the door to lasting change.

Cravings aren't defeat—they're signs that your brain is healing. Recognizing triggers and installing new habits is the key to breaking free.

Quick Win: Decode Your Triggers

1. Think of the last time you drank (or indulged in any habit you want to break)

2. Identify the trigger (stress, boredom, loneliness, celebration, etc.)

3. Ask: "What was I hoping to get?" (relief, escape, excitement, etc.)

4. Now find a healthier alternative that delivers the same feeling minus the crash

Write it down. Recognizing these triggers is step one in rewiring them.

Your #Momhak365 Challenge: Hack Your Dopamine System

Over the next 24 hours, **track every "pleasure moment"** you experience:

- Each time something feels good—your coffee, a laugh, a workout—rate it from 1–10.

- Compare if these natural pleasures feel as rewarding as they did previously.

- Notice if certain times or activities feel dull—potential areas where your dopamine system is out of sync.

Bonus: Share a natural pleasure that you rediscover today using **#Momhak365**. Collective inspiration is powerful!

Mindful Moment: Reprogramming Your Reward System

1. Close your eyes. Inhale for 4, then exhale for 6.

2. Envision your brain as a series of paths in a dense forest.

3. Each drink or destructive habit deepens the worn trail.

4. Each healthy choice forges a new path.

5. Ask yourself: "Which new trail am I creating today?"

Looking Ahead: Your Brain's Reset Button

In Chapter 3, we'll dive into:

- The Four Pillars of The Momhak Method: how to rewire cravings with Mind Hacking, Cold Exposure, Breathwork, and Moving Meditation

- The "dopamine detox" experiment and how it'll reset your pleasure system

- Immediate tools to take control instead of relying on willpower

Turn the page—your neural "operating system" awaits its next update.

CHAPTER 3: QUICKSTART TO THE MOMHAK METHOD

WHAT YOU'LL DISCOVER

- The four core pillars of The Momhak Method and how they work together
- How to reset your brain's reward system via a "dopamine detox"
- Why layering different techniques leads to stronger, lasting change
- The importance of small, consistent habits over time

KEY INSIGHTS

- Addiction rewires the brain, but **neuroplasticity** lets you rewire it back to where it was
- Mind Hacking, Mindful Breathing, Moving Meditation, and Cold Exposure each serve a unique role
- Combining these tools accelerates transformation and sustainability
- Starting small is crucial—consistency outperforms intensity

YOUR TRANSFORMATION TOOLS

- **Dopamine Detox**: Break free from artificial highs and reset your natural pleasure
- **The Four Pillars**: Mind Hacking, Cold Exposure, Mindful Breathing, and Moving Meditation

- **The Synergy Effect**: Layering techniques to reinforce positive change

- **Immediate Action**: A 15-second cold shower or 30-second breathing exercise

"We are what we repeatedly do. Excellence, then, is not an act, but a habit."
—Aristotle

From Insight to Action

In Chapters 1 and 2, we explored the emotional catalyst for change (Casey's story) and the scientific foundations of addiction and recovery (the dopamine hijack, neuroplasticity, and affirmations). Now it's time to roll up our sleeves and put theory into action. This chapter introduces the **four main pillars of The Momhak Method**—Mind Hacking, Cold Exposure, Mindful Breathing, and Moving Meditation. Think of these pillars as your core toolkit: each addresses a different aspect of your physical and mental well-being, all working together to **rewire your brain**, **reset your cravings**, and **rebuild a more resilient, purposeful life**.

A Note on the Journey Ahead

The Momhak Method isn't a "quick fix." Each pillar can dramatically shape your inner landscape, but true transformation requires **consistent practice**. As you read on, look for how these elements seamlessly integrate into daily routines, guiding you toward genuine freedom from addiction or any mental struggles you're facing. (For a step-by-step plan on applying these pillars daily, see the **Momhak 365 Challenge** in the Appendix.)

"Imagination is everything. It is the preview of life's coming attractions."
—Albert Einstein

Your Personal Power Affirmation: A Mental Reset Tool

Transforming your habits starts with transforming your identity. One of the most powerful ways to reinforce your new path is through your **Personal Power Affirmation**, first mentioned back in the Introduction. This isn't just positive thinking; it's an active rewiring of your subconscious mind.

Each time you repeat your **Personal Power Affirmation**, you signal to your brain that this is your **new reality**. Over time, these statements shift from something you *say* to something you *embody*.

If you haven't already created one, try this:
"I am strong, clear-headed, and in control. I thrive in sobriety and embrace the life I am building."

Write your affirmation down. Say it out loud in the morning. Pair it with breathwork, movement, or cold exposure. Let it **anchor you** as you move forward.

The Dopamine Reset: Preparing Your Brain

Before diving into the Four Pillars, let's address a hidden obstacle: **dopamine overload**. Addiction hijacks your reward system, making ordinary pleasures feel dull. When you're used to artificial dopamine spikes from alcohol, social media, or junk food, you might find simple rewards—like a morning walk or stretching—underwhelming. This is because your brain is still **wired for shortcuts**. Think of it like resetting your palate: If you've gotten used to processed foods that are high in sugar, salt, and oil, fresh vegetables might taste bland at first—but only until your taste buds recalibrate to appreciate natural flavors again.

How to Do a Simple Dopamine Detox

Step 1: Identify Your Biggest Dopamine Triggers

Pause and reflect: What do you turn to when stressed, bored, or uneasy? Common dopamine traps include:

- Alcohol

- Excessive caffeine

- THC

- Nicotine (cigarettes, vaping)

- Stimulants (cocaine, amphetamines)

- Opioids (heroin, prescription painkillers)

- Social media scrolling

- Binge-watching TV or gaming

- Junk food/processed sugar

- Compulsive online shopping

- Constant background noise (podcasts, music)

- News or content "doom scrolling"

- Gambling or games with chance-based rewards

- Dating apps and swiping culture

- Pornography

- Constantly checking email/messages/notifications

- Late-night internet rabbit holes

- Drama and gossip-seeking

- Mindless smartphone games

- Excessive use of delivery apps instead of cooking

- Impulsive texting or posting for validation

- "Rage-bait" content that triggers emotional responses

- Endlessly researching products without buying

- Self-medication with OTC medicines

- Obsessive stat-checking (fitness trackers, analytics)

- Extreme thrill-seeking activities

- Reflexively reaching for phone during any idle moment

Not all of these are harmful in moderation, but if they **dominate your reward system**, they block your capacity to enjoy small natural pleasures and achieve genuine, sustainable fulfillment.

Step 2: Take a 24 to 48 Hour Break

For the next one or two days, try **cutting out** your biggest artificial dopamine sources, and replace them with healthier dopamine-boosting activities:

- Move your body (yoga, hiking, or lifting weights)

- Practice breathwork (4–6 breathing, Wim Hof)

- Spend time in nature

- Read, journal, or meditate

- Engage in creative work (art, writing, music)

- Have deeper, in-person conversations

Your brain may resist—boredom or restlessness might spike, but that's a sign that it's adjusting.

Step 3: Notice the Shift

After your dopamine reset:

- Your mind feels clearer

- Small joys—a morning walk, a friendly chat—feel more rewarding

- You experience a greater sense of control over cravings

You're teaching your brain to **crave authentic fulfillment** instead of empty stimulation.

Remember, though: This isn't about banning everything forever—it's about **recalibrating your reward system**. Once you've detoxed, reintroduce technology or treats in a mindful way so that they don't control you.

Diaphragmatic Breathing: The Foundation of Breath Control

Also known as belly breathing or deep breathing, diaphragmatic breathing is one of the most effective ways to activate the parasympathetic nervous system, reduce stress, and improve oxygen efficiency. It's an essential skill for Moving Meditation, breathwork practices, and addiction recovery because it **helps regulate emotions, reduces cravings,** and **creates a sense of calm**.

How to Perform Diaphragmatic Breathing

1. **Find a Comfortable Position:** Sit or lie down in a relaxed position, placing one hand on your chest and one hand on your belly.

2. **Inhale Deeply Through Your Nose:** Breathe in slowly for around 4 to 6 seconds, allowing your belly to expand. The hand on your chest should remain still while the hand on your belly rises.

3. **Exhale Slowly Through Your Mouth:** Let the breath out gently for 6 to 8 seconds, feeling your belly fall.

4. **Repeat for 5 to 10 Minutes:** Focus on slow, controlled breaths, ensuring that your belly, not your chest, is moving.

Why It Works

- **Activates the Vagus Nerve**: Signals the brain to enter a relaxed state, reducing stress hormones.

- **Increases Oxygen Efficiency**: More oxygen reaches the brain and muscles, improving mental clarity and energy.

- **Balances the Nervous System**: Shifts from the **fight-or-flight response** (sympathetic nervous system) to **rest-and-digest mode** (parasympathetic nervous system).

- **Reduces Cravings & Anxiety**: Helps manage emotional triggers that lead to impulsive behaviors.

Integrating Diaphragmatic Breathing Into Your Daily Practice

Morning Routine: Start your day with 5 minutes of belly breathing to set a calm and focused tone.

During Cravings: When an urge arises, practice **4–6 breathing** with deep diaphragmatic engagement to regain control.

Before Sleep: Engage in 5 to 10 minutes of deep breathing to help transition into a restful state.

During Movement: Synchronize diaphragmatic breathing with **yoga, Qi Gong,** or **mindful walking** to enhance presence and relaxation.

Immediate Micro-Exercise: Diaphragmatic Breathing for Reset

Let's put diaphragmatic breathing into practice right now by following these steps:

1. Sit comfortably and place one hand on your belly and one on your chest.

2. Breathe in deeply through your nose for a slow count of 4, feeling your belly rise.

3. Exhale through your mouth for a slow count of 6, feeling your belly fall.

4. Repeat for 5 cycles, noting how your body and mind shift.

Why It Works: This exercise is a **quick nervous system reset**, ideal for stress management, reducing cravings, and maintaining emotional balance throughout the day.

"Getting sober was one of the three pivotal moments in my life, along with becoming an actor and having a child."
—Gary Oldman

The Four Pillars of The Momhak Method

Each pillar addresses a unique aspect of your mind-body system. Combined, they create **sustainable change** far more quickly than any single approach.

1. Mind Hacking (Reprogram Your Thoughts)

What It Does: Disrupts negative thought loops and installs empowering beliefs.

Techniques: Affirmations, cognitive reframing, Pain-Pleasure reset, visualization.

How to Start: Repeat your Personal Power Affirmation throughout the day (e.g., "I am in control of my mind and body, and I am thriving in sobriety.")

2. Cold Exposure (Reset Dopamine and Build Resilience)

What It Does: Trains your nervous system to handle stress without panic.

Techniques: Cold showers, face dunks, ice baths.

How to Start: In the middle of today's shower, try a **15-second blast** of cold water. Increase by 5 to 10 seconds daily.

Success Story: Many people report that consistent cold showers help reduce cravings, improve mood, and boost energy, which can make sobriety much easier.

3. Mindful Breathing (Regulate Emotions, Reduce Cravings)

What It Does: Activates the parasympathetic nervous system, lowering stress.

Techniques: 4–6 breathing, 4–7–8 breathing, Wim Hof method.

How to Start: Try **4–6 breathing** for one minute: Inhale for 4, exhale for 6.

Studies show that controlled breathing techniques, such as slow diaphragmatic breathing, can lower physiological markers of stress and improve emotional regulation, which can help reduce cravings associated with substance use disorders (Hopper et al., 2019; Perciavalle et al., 2017).

4. Moving Meditation (Anchor Yourself in the Present)

What It Does: Synchronizes mind and body, reducing cravings and stress.

Techniques: Mindful walking, Tai Chi, yoga, Qi Gong.

How to Start: Take a **5-minute mindful walk**, focusing on every step and breath.

Momhak Moment: Your Pillar Priority

Which of the Four Pillars feels most important for you right now? Write one small action you can take today using that pillar to support your recovery and growth.

The 4 Pillars of The Momhak Method & Their Core Benefits

MIND HACKING	COLD EXPOSURE	MINDFUL BREATHING	MOVING MEDITATION
Rewire your inner dialogue to break negative thought loops and build empowering beliefs that support lasting change	Reset your dopamine system and train your body to handle stress with calm resilience	Activate your parasympathetic nervous system to reduce cravings, calm anxiety, and restore emotional balance	Synchronize breath and movement to anchor your awareness in the present and reconnect mind and body

Integrate all four pillars for maximum transformation

As you start experimenting with the Four Pillars, remember: This isn't about perfection. It might feel awkward initially, but seeing others share their journey and small successes—maybe their first full minute of cold exposure or a successfully navigated craving posted with **#Momhak365**—can provide real-world encouragement. You can also find guided tutorials and shared experiences at **Momhak.com**.

Synergy: How the Four Pillars Work Together

Picture these Four Pillars as table legs—remove one, and the table wobbles. But keep them all, and you gain a **solid** foundation for transformation.

The Science of Synergy

Integrating multiple therapeutic approaches can lead to more profound and lasting transformations than relying on a single method. This concept is akin to cross-training in athletics, in which athletes combine strength, cardio, and flexibility training to achieve optimal performance. Similarly, The Momhak Method synergistically layers the Four Pillars to facilitate holistic change.

How the Pillars Strengthen Each Other

1. Mind Hacking + Cold Exposure

Integration: Pairing affirmations with the physical stimulus of Cold Exposure.

Application: Repeating "I am strong and resilient" while stepping into cold water fosters both mental and physical resilience.

2. Cold Exposure + Mindful Breathing

Integration: Using controlled breathing techniques during Cold Exposure to maintain calmness.

Application: Cold triggers the fight-or-flight response, while Mindful Breathing helps regulate this response, teaching the system to remain calm and stable under pressure.

3. Mindful Breathing + Moving Meditation

Integration: Combining breath focus with physical movement practices like yoga or Qi Gong.

Application: Coordinating breath with movement deepens both practices, enhancing focus and reinforcing the mind-body connection.

4. Moving Meditation + Mind Hacking

Integration: Incorporating affirmations into physical movement.

Application: Chanting a key phrase while walking strengthens the mind-body connection for a deeper impact.

By weaving these practices together, The Momhak Method creates a comprehensive framework that addresses multiple facets of well-being, leading to a more robust and enduring transformation.

The Recovery Advantage

When cravings arise, you have multiple tools at your disposal:

1. Mindful Breathing to calm your nerves

2. Mind Hacking to reframe the situation

3. Cold shower to reset your system

4. Moving Meditation to process emotions

Rather than relying on one "silver bullet," you can **layer** these approaches for maximum effect.

Safety & Precautions

Before integrating these pillars, keep the following in mind:

Medical Conditions: If you have heart problems, respiratory issues, or any chronic health concerns, consult a physician before trying cold showers, extended breath holds, or vigorous movement.

Gentle Start: Ease into the pillars. The Momhak Method is about sustainable, long-term change—it's shouldn't be an extreme shock that leaves you discouraged or injured.

Listen to Your Body: Discomfort can be productive, but pain signals a need to stop or modify. Pay close attention to fatigue, dizziness, or shortness of breath.

Remember: Progress gradually. If 15 seconds of cold water feels intense, that's okay. Consistency trumps intensity. You want to build a routine that you can maintain for the long haul.

Immediate Micro-Exercise: The 15-Second Cold Shower

Let's put the Cold Exposure pillar into practice right now—or, more precisely, during your next shower. After washing with warm water, turn the dial to cold for just **15 seconds**. After the icy blast, feel free to turn the water back to warm. Stay calm, breathe steadily, and notice the following:

Breathing Focus: Resist the urge to hyperventilate—just try to relax and breathe normally.

Mental Check-In: Observe the initial shock. Remind yourself, "This is temporary and I'm safe."

Write It Down: Afterward, jot down how you felt—both physically and mentally.

Why It Works: Doing something uncomfortable but safe rewires your response to stress. You train your brain that short-term discomfort can lead to a long-term reward: resilience, mental clarity, and a natural dopamine boost.

Optional Next Step: Over the next week, gradually increase the cold-water exposure by 5- to 10-second increments. Notice how each small step builds confidence and grit.

Overcoming Initial Resistance

It's natural to feel some reluctance about cold showers, daily movement, or confronting negative thoughts. Let's look at a few strategies below to help you push past your initial barriers.

Focus on Benefits: Instead of dwelling on discomfort, remind yourself of the payoff—clearer thinking, better mood, and less reliance on substances.

Start Small: If 15 seconds of cold water is too much, try 5 seconds. If you can't manage a full yoga session, do 2 or 3 simple stretches. Progress at your own pace.

Accountability: Share your plan with a friend or a support group. Knowing that someone is cheering you on (or asking how your practice went) can give you the extra nudge you need.

Mental Reframe

The pillars aren't punishments—they're gifts. They offer a natural high, a sense of mastery, and a path to freedom from the treadmill of addiction.

Practical Tips & Troubleshooting

1. Mind Hacking Obstacles

Common Challenge: "I've tried affirmations but they feel fake."

Solution: Adjust your language. If "I'm unstoppable" feels too grandiose, try "I'm learning to be stronger each day." Authenticity matters for affirmations to resonate.

2. Cold Exposure Nuances

Common Challenge: Cold water is too painful, or you're feeling panicked.

Solution: Make the water temperature cool rather than ice-cold to start. Focus on **slow, calm breathing** throughout the exposure, then gradually decrease the water temperature over time.

3. Mindful Breathing Hurdles

Common Challenge: Mind wandering or boredom.

Solution: Instead of fighting wandering thoughts, gently acknowledge them and redirect attention to the breath, without judgment. Consider setting a timer for just one minute initially.

4. Moving Meditation Problems

Common Challenge: Lack of space or privacy.

Solution: Even a corner of your bedroom can work for a brief yoga flow or a few standing Chi Gong exercises. Some movements can also be done seated in a chair, focusing on upper body flow if standing space is limited.

Remember: The goal here isn't perfection; each pillar is an ongoing practice that evolves as you grow. Take note of your progress in a journal or daily planner to spot improvements over time (see the Appendix for the **Momhak 365 Challenge**).

Mind Hacking in Action: A Quick Mini-Exercise

Morning Reframe:

1. **Identify one negative thought** you've had about your sobriety or mental health in the past 24 hours. Example: *I'm too weak to resist cravings.*

2. **Question & Replace:** Ask yourself, *Is this 100% true?* Usually, it isn't. Then replace it with a more balanced statement: *I'm learning to handle cravings, and each urge I overcome makes me stronger.*

Affirm & Feel: Speak your new statement out loud or write it in your journal. Take a moment to let it sink in—feel the relief, hope, or determination it sparks.

Short Summary of What's Ahead

Now that you've learned about the Four Pillars, you're ready to see how they weave through the entire Momhak Method going forward.

Chapters 4 & 5: We'll dive deeper into Cold Exposure and Moving Meditation, guiding you from 15-second cold showers to longer, more invigorating practices—and from simple, mindful movement to sequences that build rhythm, resilience, and presence. I'll also share real-life stories of people just like you who've overcome anxiety, cravings, and stress with these practices.

Chapter 6: We'll explore Mind Hacking—the art of rewiring your thoughts and beliefs to support lasting change. You'll learn how to break old patterns using affirmations, visualization, and the pain–pleasure principle, installing new beliefs that align with your growth and recovery.

Chapters 7: Daily habit-building—learning how to reframe negative thoughts and integrate healthy behaviors (like better nutrition and improved sleep) into your routine.

Chapters 8 & 9: We'll tackle social triggers, boundary-setting, and finding deeper purpose. You'll learn how to handle parties, family gatherings, or tough days without turning to a drink or other substance. We will also look deeper into the role THC can play in helping, hindering, or becoming an addiction of its own.

Chapter 10: Finally, we'll expand beyond sobriety to explore living a vibrant, purpose-driven life. Think of it as your blueprint for *thriving*, not just surviving.

Where We're Headed: The intent isn't just to remove alcohol or substances from your life—it's also to fill that space with a new sense of empowerment, purpose, and healthy brain chemistry. By mastering the Four Pillars, you're laying the foundation for everything that comes next.

Chapter 3 Summary: QuickStart to the Momhak Method

Core Message

Your brain can be rewired—and The Momhak Method is your blueprint. Small, consistent actions—not willpower alone—create lasting change.

Key Lessons

Addiction isn't just mental—it's also physical. Your brain's dopamine system needs a reset, and that reset starts with action.

The Four Pillars each address a different angle of recovery: Mind Hacking, Cold Exposure, Mindful Breathing, and Moving Meditation.

Starting small is the key to long-term success. Consistency beats intensity. Tiny shifts, repeated daily, will transform your life.

Your #Momhak365 Challenge: Pick One Pillar to Try

Pick one of the Four Pillars and practice it for 30 seconds:

Mind Hacking: Speak your Personal Power Affirmation out loud (e.g., "I'm strong, clear-headed, and in control.").

Cold Exposure: Try a blast of cold water in the middle of your shower.

Mindful Breathing: Try 4–6 breathing (inhale for 4 seconds, exhale for 6 seconds) for 3 rounds.

Moving Meditation: Take a slow, mindful walk, or do 5 minutes of gentle stretching.

Notice how you feel. A small shift now paves a new neural path.

Bonus: Share your experience using **#Momhak365**. Inspire others by showing how easy it is to begin.

Mindful Moment: The Compound Effect of Small Actions

1. Close your eyes. Inhale for 4, exhale for 6.

2. Visualize each small action as a drop of water on a dry sponge.

3. Initially, the sponge is rigid. But with each drop, it softens and transforms.

4. Your daily micro-habits are these drops, reshaping your brain over time.

You don't need massive change right now—just **one** drop. Which drop will you choose today?

Looking Ahead: The Physical Reset

In Chapter 4, we'll **dive deeper** into Cold Exposure and Mindful Breathing, exploring:

• How cold therapy elevates dopamine and resilience

• Specific breathing techniques for stress and craving rewiring

• Why these tools often outperform sheer willpower

Go ahead—step into the cold. Your next breakthrough awaits.

CHAPTER 4: THE PHYSICAL RESET

WHAT YOU'LL DISCOVER

- How Cold Exposure and Mindful Breathing reset your nervous system

- The science behind dopamine, stress resilience, and immune benefits

- Why physical and mental interventions are equally vital in recovery

- How to integrate cold therapy and breathing into daily life

KEY INSIGHTS

- Cold Exposure naturally boosts dopamine, thus reducing cravings

- Breathwork helps regulate emotions and stress, which makes relapse less likely

- Combined, they build mental and physical resilience

- Small, consistent exposure works better than extreme methods

YOUR TRANSFORMATION TOOLS

- Cold Exposure Progression: From cold showers to ice baths

- Breathing Techniques: 4–6 Breathing, 4–7–8, Tummo/Wim Hof

- Tracking & Habit Stacking: Making these practices stick

- Hormesis: Using small stressors to cultivate long-term resilience

"The mind and the body are two sides of the same coin; transforming one often requires tending to the other."
—Unknown

The First Cold Shower: Facing the Mind's Resistance

The first time I turned my shower dial to ice cold, every instinct screamed, "No!"—my breath seized, my muscles tensed, and my mind begged me to jump out. I'd spent years avoiding discomfort by drinking to numb stress and escaping into bad habits whenever life got tough. Now, under freezing water, I was doing the exact opposite: letting discomfort happen *on purpose*.

Those opening seconds were brutal. Panic rose—my body fought the cold, just like my mind had once fought cravings and negative thoughts. Then I did something different: I **breathed**. A deep inhale, then a slow exhale, relaxing my shoulders. The cold remained, but something shifted—it no longer **controlled** me.

As I stepped out, I felt electrified. It was like I'd conquered a battle against myself—and in many ways, I had. I realized that if I could train my nervous system to stay calm in the cold, I could train it to stay calm under cravings and stress. This wasn't just an exercise in willpower—it was a **reset** for my mind and body.

A Call to Action

If you're ready, commit to the **#Momhak365 Challenge**—a 30-day **Cold Exposure + Mindful Breathing reset** designed to rewire your stress response and bolster resilience. You'll find a full outline later in the chapter and in the appendix, but why wait? Start today with a 15-second cold rinse and a simple breathwork session. Track how you feel and share your progress with **#Momhak365**.

Why Focus on the Physical?

Many recovery programs emphasize mental and emotional work—and rightfully so. But what we often underestimate is **the power of the body in rewiring the mind**. Cold Exposure and Mindful Breathing are more than just "hacks"—they're physiological resets that can elevate mood, reduce cravings, and build the resilience needed for lasting transformation. In this chapter, we'll explore how **intentional cold exposure and controlled breathwork can rewire your nervous system**, helping you handle stress, break addictive cycles, and cultivate a stronger, calmer mind.

> *"Discomfort is the price of admission to a meaningful life."*
> —Susan David, Harvard psychologist and author of *Emotional Agility*

Deep Dive on Cold Exposure

Why Cold Therapy?

For many people, the idea of plunging into icy water or taking a cold shower sounds like a mild form of torture, but both **modern research** and **ancient traditions** reveal something remarkable: **Controlled Cold Exposure offers profound benefits**. From **boosting dopamine** and norepinephrine to **strengthening stress resilience and immune function**, Cold Exposure trains both your mind and body to **handle discomfort**—an essential skill for breaking addictive cycles. Let's break down why this uncomfortable act can be a game-changer in your transformation.

Dopamine & Norepinephrine Boost

- A 2000 study found that cold water immersion (at 57°F/14°C) for one hour increased norepinephrine levels by 530% and dopamine by 250% (Srámek et al. 2000).

- These chemicals help regulate mood, reduce cravings, and increase alertness, making them a powerful tool for addiction recovery.

Mood Elevation & Stress Resilience

- Exposing your body to cold teaches your nervous system to **stay calm under pressure**—a concept called stress inoculation.

- By learning to breathe through discomfort, you build emotional and physical resilience, making you less reactive to everyday stressors.

- Cold showers and plunges **lower cortisol (the stress hormone)** and activate the parasympathetic nervous system, leaving you feeling **calm yet energized**.

Metabolic Activation & Fat Regulation

- Cold Exposure forces your body to work harder to stay warm, **increasing calorie burn.**

- It activates brown adipose tissue (BAT)—a type of fat that burns energy to generate heat, helping with insulin sensitivity and metabolic regulation (van Marken Lichtenbelt & Schrauwen, 2011).

- While not a magic bullet for weight loss, regular Cold Exposure supports metabolic function and enhances overall energy levels.

Immune Support

- Cold Exposure (combined with breathwork) has been shown to **enhance immune function** (Kox et al., 2014).

- Practitioners, including myself, often report **fewer common illnesses**, possibly due to higher white blood cell counts.

A Word on Hormesis

The concept of hormesis says that small amounts of controlled stress make you stronger over time. Just like lifting weights strengthens your muscles, short-term exposure to cold trains your nervous system to be more resilient to stress, cravings, and emotional turbulence.

This is why Cold Exposure is more than just a biohacking trend—it's a proven physiological tool for rewiring how your mind and body respond to discomfort.

Case Study: Raúl (Multi-Substance Addiction)

For years, Raúl bounced among recovery programs with minimal success. Craving a new approach, he discovered the Wim Hof Method—combining deep breathing and daily cold showers. Within weeks, he felt unprecedented control over cravings and emotional swings. "It saved my life," he says, and now consistently uses breathwork and Cold Exposure as a daily mental reset (Carney, 2017).

"The Ice Man" Wim Hof

The transformative power of Cold Exposure and Mindful Breathing is exemplified in the journey of Wim Hof, known as "The Iceman" for his extraordinary feats in extreme cold. In 1995, Hof faced profound personal tragedy when his wife, Olaya, committed suicide, leaving him to care for their four children. Struggling with overwhelming grief and searching for a way to cope, Hof turned to the cold. Immersing himself in freezing water, he discovered that the intense sensation provided a respite from his mental anguish, allowing him to find clarity and resilience.

This practice not only helped him navigate his loss but also led to the development of the Wim Hof Method, a combination of Cold Exposure, specific breathing techniques, and meditation. Hof's technique has since gained global recognition, with practitioners reporting benefits such as increased stress tolerance, enhanced immune response, and improved mental health. His journey underscores the potential of these practices to facilitate profound personal transformation, even in the face of life's most challenging circumstances (Carney 2017).

What Doesn't Kill Us

The impact of Cold Exposure and Mindful Breathing extends beyond its originator, resonating with individuals worldwide. One notable example is investigative journalist and anthropologist Scott Carney. Initially approaching Wim Hof's methods with skepticism, Carney aimed to debunk what he presumed were exaggerated claims. But upon immersing himself in the practices, his perspective shifted dramatically.

In his 2017 book *What Doesn't Kill Us*, Carney recounts his transformative journey. He describes how, under Hof's guidance, he undertook challenges that seemed insurmountable, such as climbing a snow-covered Mount Kilimanjaro wearing minimal clothing. Through consistent practice of controlled breathing and gradual Cold Exposure, Carney experienced enhanced physical endurance, mental clarity, and a profound sense of resilience. His journey from skeptic to believer highlights how cold therapy and breathwork can reveal latent capacities—which is beneficial for anyone seeking physical or mental growth, including those recovering from addiction.

Ancient Traditions of Cold-Water Strengthening

While Wim Hof has popularized modern Cold Exposure, he's far from the first to discover its power. For centuries, cultures around the world have used cold water as a tool for purification, resilience, and spiritual growth. Let's examine some of them below.

Samurai & Misogi: The Cold Path to Clarity

In Japan, **misogi** is a Shinto purification ritual in which individuals immerse themselves in icy waterfalls or cold rivers to cleanse their bodies and minds. Practitioners believe that the cold water washes away negative energy and restores their connection to nature. While not exclusive to the samurai, a related practice known as **Takigyo**—the ritual of standing beneath a cold waterfall—was sometimes used by warriors and monks alike to cultivate **mental discipline, emotional control,** and **spiritual resilience**. Enduring the sting of ice-cold water wasn't just a test of the body; it was a test of the will, a way to train the nervous system to remain calm in chaos—a principle deeply aligned with Bushido, the samurai code of honor and courage.

Even today, martial artists, monks, and spiritual seekers continue this ancient tradition. They don't do it for comfort—they do it to awaken something deeper. Each drop of cold water becomes a teacher. Each breath taken in the midst of discomfort becomes a doorway to presence.

Like Cold Exposure in The Momhak Method, misogi is more than a challenge—it's a ceremony of self-overcoming. A reminder that when you face discomfort directly, you don't just survive it—you transform through it.

Haida & Makah Cold-Water Rituals (Pacific Northwest First Nations)

Among the Indigenous peoples of the Pacific Northwest, cold-water immersion has long served as a means of spiritual purification, physical resilience, and connection to the natural world.

Haida Nation: Ocean as Healer

For the Haida people of Haida Gwaii, the ocean is more than sustenance—it's *sacred*. Practices like ocean bathing and saltwater cleansing are used to purify the body, mind, and spirit. These rituals are believed to wash away negative energy and restore balance, reinforcing the sacred relationship between humans and the sea.

Makah Tribe: Rituals of Readiness

The Makah tribe of Neah Bay, Washington, have long prepared for whale hunts with rigorous spiritual and physical conditioning. This includes fasting, isolation, and ceremonial cold-water immersion. Such practices are integral to ensuring that hunters are in the right mental and physical state to honor the spirit of the whale they pursue.

For these cultures, Cold Exposure transcends mere endurance—it's also a pathway to align with nature, sharpen instincts, and cultivate profound inner strength.

Beginner vs. Advanced Protocols

Beginner: If you're new to cold showers, start with 10 to 15 seconds of cold water in the middle of your usual warm shower. Gradually increase to 30 seconds, then a minute (or more). Experiment with this at the beginning, middle, and end of your shower. I prefer to begin with a 2- to 3-minute cold shower to invigorate my system, followed by a warm, lingering shower to relax my muscles and promote blood flow.

Intermediate: Once you can handle a 1- to 2-minute cold shower with relative ease, consider exploring cold plunges. Aim for water between 50 and 60°F (10 and 15°C) to experience benefits without overwhelming your system.

Advanced: True "cold plunges" or winter swimming can push water temperatures below 50°F (10°C). Approach these extremes with caution, thorough preparation, and possibly under the guidance of an experienced mentor.

Safety & Best Practices

Check Your Health Status: If you have cardiovascular issues, high blood pressure, or other chronic health problems, consult with a medical professional before plunging into cold therapy.

Mindset Matters: Rather than bracing for the experience with fear, approach the cold with curiosity. Slow, Mindful Breathing as you enter cold water can significantly reduce the shock factor.

Track Your Tolerance: Each body is unique. Use a journal or app to note the water temperature and duration, as well as how you felt afterward.

> *"If you want to conquer the anxiety of life, live in the moment, live in the breath."*
> —Amit Ray, author and meditation teacher

Breathing Techniques

Few tools are as universally accessible as the breath. We do it constantly and yet seldom pay attention to how it shapes our emotional and physical state. In this section, we'll explore three core methods: 4–6 Breathing, 4–7–8 Breathing, and Tummo/Wim Hof Breathing.

4–6 Breathing

How: Inhale through your nose for a count of 4, then exhale for 6.
Why: The prolonged extended exhale activates the parasympathetic nervous system, lowering stress hormones like cortisol and shifting you from fight-or-flight to rest-and-digest (Brown & Gerbarg, 2009).
When: It's perfect for quick stress relief during traffic jams, mini-breaks, or pre-sleep calm.

4–7–8 Breathing

How: Inhale through your nose for 4 seconds, hold for 7, then exhale for 8.
Why: This technique can swiftly reduce anxiety, making it a favorite among insomniacs seeking calm before bed. By increasing

the exhale time and adding a breath-hold, you deepen the relaxation effect.

Contraindications: If extended breath holds feel uncomfortable, shorten the hold time. Always listen to your body's cues.

Tummo/Wim Hof Breathing

Origins: A Tibetan Buddhist practice popularized by Wim Hof.
How:

- Lie down in a safe environment (never while driving or immersed in water).

- Take 30 deep, rhythmic breaths, fully inhaling and letting each exhale flow naturally.

- After the last breath, exhale about 90% and hold until you feel discomfort.

- Inhale fully, hold for 10 to 15 seconds, then release.

- Repeat for 3 rounds.

Why:

- **Boosts Immune Response:** In one clinical trial, participants using Wim Hof breathing plus Cold Exposure showed reduced inflammatory markers when exposed to an endotoxin (Kox et al., 2014).

- **Stress Adaptation:** Regulates the body's response to external stressors, teaching the mind to stay calm in high-stress situations.

- **Energy & Focus:** Tummo breathing can lead to a "clean" surge of energy, clarity, and potentially higher oxygen saturation.

- **Mood Lift:** Many practitioners—including myself—report a noticeable elevation in mood for hours after a session.

Safety: If you feel dizzy or faint, stop. Never combine breath holds with driving or swimming.

I practice Wim Hof breathing **first thing in the morning while still in bed**, and it's completely changed how I start my day. The rush of oxygen wakes me up naturally, giving me an immediate **boost of energy, focus, and mental clarity**. It used to be a struggle to get out of bed, but now, after just a few rounds of breathwork, I feel fully awake and ready to take on the day. I also use the breath-hold phase to repeat affirmations, combining two powerful techniques into one practice. By doing this, I not only supercharge my energy levels but also reprogram my mindset, setting a strong, positive tone for the day ahead.

Core Breathing Techniques

4–6 BREATHING	4-7-8 BREATHNG	TUMMO / WIM HOF BREATHING
• Inhale: 4 seconds • Exhale: 6 seconds • **Benefits:** Quick stress relief, parasympathetic activation • **When to use:** Anytime, especially during cravings or anxiety	• Inhale: 4 seconds • Hold: 7 seconds • Exhale: 8 seconds • **Benefits:** Deeper relaxation, enhanced sleep, nervous system regulation • **When to use:** Before bed, during heightened stress	• 30-40 deep, rhythmic breaths • Final exhale and hold until urge to breathe • Deep inhale, 15-second hold, release • Do 2-3 rounds for maximum benefit • **When to use:** Morning, miday or evening

Feel the Breath: Wherever you are, stop and practice just **three** full cycles of the 4–6 breathing technique. Don't just do it; **feel it**. Notice the rise and fall of your abdomen, the temperature of the air, and the pause between breaths.

Weekly Schedule & Tracking

Consistency cements these new habits. The following is a **7-day plan** to incrementally scale Cold Exposure and Mindful Breathing. Feel free to modify as you see fit.

Day	Cold Exposure	Breathing Practice	Notes/Journal
1	15-second cold shower	5 rounds of 4–6 breathing (morning)	Post-shower mood/energy
2	20-second cold shower	1 or 2 rounds of Tummo/Wim Hof, affirmations during breath holds	Track your breath holds. Which felt easiest?
3	25-second cold shower	4–7–8 breathing before bed (5 rounds)	Rate your sleep quality the next morning
4	30-second cold shower	2 or 3 Tummo rounds daily; affirmations during breath holds	Any emotional shifts? More or fewer cravings?
5	35-second cold shower	5 rounds of 4–6 midday or under stress	Observe dips in your energy or stress
6	40-second cold shower	3 Tummo rounds (morning) + 4–7–8 (night)	Compare your morning vs. night mental states
7	40- to 60-second cold shower	Choose any combo of technique + affirmations	Evaluate. Which approach resonates most?

Reflection: Note changes in your mood, cravings, energy, and sleep. This helps you spot what's most beneficial.

Overcoming Resistance

No matter how promising a habit, **resistance** often appears. Let's examine some common roadblocks and strategies to conquer them:

"I hate the cold!"

- **Mindset Shift:** Discomfort can be a catalyst for growth. Start small—just 10 seconds—then increase.

- **Reward System:** Promise yourself a positive ritual afterward, like a calming herbal tea or reading a few lines of an inspiring book.

"I don't have time!"

- **Habit Stacking:** Pair your breathing practice with **affirmations** when making coffee or another routine task. For instance, immediately after brushing your teeth or before opening your laptop, do a round of 4–6 breathing with your Personal Power Affirmation or other positive statement: "I am steady, I am strong."

- **Plan for Success:** Keep a mental or physical checklist. Each day you manage even a brief practice, mark it off. The visible progress can be highly motivating.

"This feels too intense!"

- **Pace Yourself:** If Wim Hof breathing or ice-cold plunges feel overwhelming, use gentler forms—like 4–6 breathing or lukewarm water. Gradual progression is key.

- **Seek Support:** Online communities exist for Cold Exposure and Mindful Breathing. Sharing experiences can normalize initial discomfort and spark new ideas.

"I tried once, but I got discouraged."

- **Celebrate Small Wins:** Even 15 seconds under cold water is a victory. Consistency builds confidence.

- **Refine, Don't Quit:** If a certain method didn't resonate, experiment with another. The Momhak Method offers multiple tools for a reason.

Combining Cold Exposure & Breathwork

Each method alone is potent; **together**, they unleash synergy beyond the sum of their parts.

Layering Techniques

1. Pre-Cold Shower Breathing:

- **Perform 2 or 3 rounds of Wim Hof or 4–6 breathing** before stepping into the shower. This can steady your mind and reduce the initial shock.

- **Focus on taking long, controlled inhales and exhales**, mentally preparing yourself for the cold.

2. In-Shower Focus:

- **As you transition to cold water, maintain slow, rhythmic breathing** rather than short, panicked breaths. This trains your nervous system to remain calm under stress.

- **Recite affirmations** during the cold shower—such as, "I'm strong enough to face discomfort," or "I welcome this challenge and will grow from it."

3. Post-Cold Recovery Breathing:

- **After the shower, continue your 4–6 breathing** to help your body transition back to its normal state.

- **Notice the tingling sensations or burst of energy**—a sign that your body is responding positively to both the cold and controlled breathing.

Momhak Moment: Full-Day Mood Boost

A morning Wim Hof breathing session and an afternoon cold shower can sustain your good mood for much of the day. By starting your morning with deep, energizing breaths, you prime your body and mind for alertness and resilience. Then in the afternoon, a brief cold shower resets your stress levels and recharges your energy—helping you avoid that mid-afternoon slump.

Why It Works

Physiological Pairing: Cold shocks the system into a heightened state, while breathing techniques modulate that response. This interplay strengthens your stress threshold.

Chemical Cascades: Both methods elevate dopamine and reduce cortisol, creating a one-two punch that can significantly stabilize mood and cravings.

Expanded Monthly Progression Plan

If you want more than a 7-day schedule, try this 30-day progression:

Week	Cold Exposure	Breathing Practice	Focus
1	10- 30-second cold shower, 3x/week	2 or 3 Tummo + affirmations daily	Get comfortable with the basics
2	30- 60-second cold shower, 4 or 5x/week	2 or 3 Tummo + affirmations daily, 4–7–8 breathing at night	Notice calmer days and stable mood; track emotional balance
3	60- 120-second cold shower, nearly daily	2 or 3 Tummo + affirmations daily,	Amplify dopamine boost; track

		4–6 breathing when stressed	emotional balance
4	60- to 120-second cold shower, daily (optional cold plunge)	3 Tummo + affirmations daily, 4–6 breathing at bedtime	Solidify routine; refine best techniques

Each Sunday, review your notes. Are certain breath exercises more helpful during cravings? Does your overall stress or sleep improve?

FAQs

Cold Exposure Questions

What if I have a heart condition or high blood pressure? Is Cold Exposure safe for me?

If you have cardiovascular conditions, always consult a doctor before attempting full cold immersion. However, gentler methods like face dunks, cold hand immersion, or a lukewarm rinse before cooling down gradually can still be beneficial. Avoid extreme shocks to your system.

I tried a cold shower, but I panicked. How do I stay calm?

The panic response is normal. Instead of forcing yourself through it, focus on your breathing first. Try 4–6 breathing before stepping in. Start small—first just your feet, then your hands, then splash cold water on your face before going full-body.

How long does it take to feel the benefits?

Many people feel an immediate boost in energy and alertness after their first cold shower. But for long-term dopamine regulation, mood improvement, and stress resilience, aim for at least two weeks of consistent practice to notice significant changes.

Can I just do cold showers without breathwork?

Yes, but combining both maximizes results. Breathwork helps control your stress response, making Cold Exposure easier. It also enhances dopamine and oxygen levels, supercharging the benefits.

Will cold showers make me sick?

No, quite the opposite. Research suggests that regular cold showers can strengthen the immune system, increasing white blood cell production. However, if you're already sick, skip the Cold Exposure and focus on breathwork to aid recovery.

Do I have to take ice baths, or are cold showers enough?

Cold showers are enough. Even just 15- to 30-seconds of cold water triggers powerful physiological benefits. Ice baths are optional for those who want a deeper reset, but consistency with cold showers is more important than extreme temperatures.

Breathwork Questions

Is holding my breath dangerous?

Breathwork is safe when done correctly. Always practice while seated or lying down, never while driving or in water. If you feel dizzy, stop and return to normal breathing.

How do I know which breathing technique to use?

It depends on your goal:

- 4–6 Breathing (inhale for 4 seconds, exhale for 6 seconds): Calming and stress reduction

- 4–7–8 Breathing (inhale for 4 seconds, hold for 7, exhale 8for): Faster sleep and anxiety relief

- Tummo/Wim Hof Method – Energizing, dopamine boost, cold resistance

Can I do breathwork at any time of day?

Yes, but some techniques have optimal timing:

- Morning: Tummo/Wim Hof for energy and focus. Avoid doing Wim Hof on a full stomach

- Midday break and when stressed: 4–6 breathing for calm and clarity

- Before bed: 4–7–8 breathing for deeper sleep

Final Thoughts: Lifelong Cold Exposure & Breathwork

Key Takeaways

Start small: Both cold showers and breath routines get easier with practice.

Consistency: A 15-second cold rinse each day beats an occasional ice bath every few weeks.

Track your progress: Journaling or habit apps help you see improvements and stay engaged.

Combine approaches for best results: Pairing Mind Hacking, breathwork, Cold Exposure, and Moving Meditation turbocharges brain rewiring.

Chapter 4 Summary: The Physical Reset

Core Message

Your body is a key player in rewiring your brain. Cold Exposure and Mindful Breathing aren't just gimmicks—they reset your nervous system, boost dopamine naturally, and build resilience.

Key Lessons

Cold Exposure elevates dopamine, reduces cravings, and stabilizes mood.

Breathwork manages stress, vital for preventing relapse.

Small, consistent practices trump extremes—daily cold showers and short breath sessions can spark major changes.

Your #Momhak365 Challenge: Cold + Breath Reset
Over the next 7 days:

- 15 seconds to 2 minutes of cold water in the middle of your shower while practicing 4–6 breathing

- 2 or 3 rounds Wim Hof breathing per day

Track how you feel. Over time, you'll see:

- Higher dopamine (less artificial reward-seeking)

- Sharper mental clarity

- Bolstered stress response

Once you've completed these first 7 days, you definitely can't stop there. You've just built the momentum—now it's time to lock in the habit. Move on to the **monthly schedule** and continue progressing. If you can complete 30 days, you'll start to see the true transformation of Cold Exposure and Mindful Breathing in your life.

Cold Exposure isn't just a solo practice—it's a movement. People all over the world are taking the **#Momhak365 challenge**, stepping into discomfort, and reshaping their minds and bodies. Track your progress, share your streak, and connect with others using **#Momhak365.** Let's build resilience together.

Looking Ahead: Moving Meditation
In Chapter 5, we'll explore **movement** and its power to rewire the brain:

- How **Tai Chi, yoga, and Chi Gong** reduce stress and boost dopamine

- The **science of flow states** and why movement can be meditation

- How to use **affirmations + movement** to reprogram negative thought patterns

CHAPTER 5: MOVING MEDITATION

WHAT YOU'LL DISCOVER

- How movement can be an accessible form of meditation
- Why practices like yoga, Tai Chi, Qi Gong, and mindful walking can rewire the brain and reduce cravings
- The link between physical motion, stress relief, and dopamine balance
- Practical methods to integrate Moving Meditation into everyday life for clarity and resilience

KEY INSIGHTS

- Sitting quietly isn't the only path—movement can be equally meditative
- Synchronizing breath with motion deepens mind-body awareness
- Gentle, rhythmic movement helps regulate emotions and decrease cravings
- Small, consistent practice leads to long-term breakthroughs

YOUR TRANSFORMATION TOOLS

- Yoga, Tai Chi, Qi Gong, and mindful walks: Simple ways to introduce mindful movement
- Micro-Practices: Short, 5-minute approaches to remaining present
- The Science of Flow: How movement shifts brain chemistry to aid recovery

- Affirmations + Movement: Embodying positive beliefs through physical action

Remember: If you have mobility or balance concerns, adapt movements accordingly. Consult a healthcare professional if you're unsure about new exercise routines.

"We don't always sit to find stillness; sometimes we move—and the stillness finds us."
—Unknown

Meditation in Motion

I always wanted to be someone who could sit in stillness for hours, effortlessly clearing my mind. And for short periods, I could. But before long, I'd find myself shifting, restless, my thoughts racing ahead. The idea of sitting still while my mind buzzed felt like trying to hold back a river with my bare hands.

As a kid, I was always moving. I grew up playing sports—running, climbing, stretching, constantly in motion. Diving was my main sport, and training for competitions meant hours of refining technique, syncing breath with movement, and visualizing each dive before I even stepped onto the board. Looking back, it was a form of meditation—I just didn't call it that at the time, of course.

Later in life, when I tried seated meditation, I struggled. The more I forced myself to be still, the more my mind resisted. It wasn't that I couldn't focus—it was that my body needed to be part of the process.

Then I had a realization—one that had been right in front of me all along. When I stretched, when I moved, when my breath synchronized with my body, my mind naturally quieted. I wasn't fighting myself anymore—I was working *with* myself.

It clicked when I started practicing Tai Chi and certain forms of yoga. The rhythmic flow of movement, the controlled breath, the way each motion required presence—it was everything I'd been looking for in meditation, just in a different form. It wasn't about shutting off my thoughts; it was about channeling them into my body, into movement, into breath.

I see meditation completely differently now. It's not about sitting still—it's about finding stillness within movement. If sitting meditation works for you, that's fantastic. But if, like me, you feel more at home when your body is engaged, know that presence isn't limited to just stillness. Some of us need to *move* to find it.

Why Movement Matters

Tolle's Emphasis on "Being in Your Body"

In *The Power of Now*, Eckhart Tolle often speaks about **"inner body awareness"** as a gateway to presence—but what if awareness isn't just about feeling the body? What if it's about **moving with it**? The mind can wander in stillness, but in motion, awareness has an anchor—the rhythm of breath, the shifting of weight, the flow of movement. Moving Meditation transforms Tolle's concept of presence from a passive state into an **active engagement with the present moment**.

Moving Meditation is a natural extension of Tolle's philosophy: By actively engaging your body through deliberate motion, you're more able to easily maintain that sliver of awareness on your bodily sensations. Your mind has less chance to spin out into worry or rumination because it's busy tracking breath and muscular changes.

Finding Clarity Through Motion

One morning after another failed attempt at seated meditation, I stood up and stretched. Instinctively, I inhaled as I reached my arms overhead and exhaled as I folded forward. My breath and body moved as one, and for the first time that morning, my mind stopped racing. There was no struggle and no force—just an effortless presence.

From that moment on, instead of fighting my nature, **I leaned into it**. My meditation became a practice of moving with awareness— Tai Chi, yoga, even walking. The more I moved, the calmer my mind became.

Training for Stillness: How Moving Meditation Prepares the Mind

Many people struggle with traditional seated meditation, finding that their thoughts become louder the moment they attempt to be still. But what if movement can be the very tool that trains the mind for stillness? Just as physical exercise builds strength for athletic performance, Moving Meditation conditions the nervous system to tolerate quiet and stillness. By engaging the body first— through Tai Chi, yoga, or mindful walking—you create a rhythm of presence that naturally extends into moments of rest. As movement and breath become familiar anchors over time, the transition into seated mindfulness feels less daunting. The ultimate goal isn't just to move mindfully—it's also to cultivate the ability to sit with yourself, in full presence, without needing distraction or escape.

Additional Moving Meditation Activities

While Tai Chi, yoga, and mindful walking are some of the most well-known forms of Moving Meditation, many other physical activities can serve the same purpose **when practiced with intention**. The key is to engage in movement that allows you to synchronize breath with motion, creating a rhythmic, meditative state. Below are some additional activities that lend themselves particularly well to Moving Meditation:

- **Hiking** – Using nature as an anchor, allow your breath to sync with the rhythm of your steps

- **Paddleboarding** – Engages balance and core strength while promoting breath awareness on water

- **Rock Climbing** – Requires deep presence and controlled breathing to navigate each movement

- **Swimming** – When done mindfully, strokes and breath align naturally into a rhythm

- **Dancing** – Free-flowing movement that allows for spontaneous presence and expression

- **Gardening** – Digging, planting, and pruning in a mindful, intentional manner

- **Cycling** – Maintaining a steady cadence while focusing on breath and movement

- **Rowing or Kayaking** – Repetitive, meditative strokes that cultivate focus and breath control

- **Jump Rope** – Done naturally and rhythmically, it creates a focused state of movement and breath

- **Skateboarding or Surfing** – Demands presence, balance, and fluid movement

- **Martial Arts** – Forms like aikido emphasize fluid, meditative motion

Mindful Movement: Amplifying the Benefits

Moving Meditation does more than improve focus—it reconfigures how we experience presence as well. Unlike seated meditation (in which awareness is primarily internal), Moving Meditation integrates mind, breath, and motion, forging a profound embodiment of the present moment.

For those who find seated meditation challenging, mindful movement channels restlessness into **purposeful action**, bridging emotional processing and physical expression.

But insight alone won't change habits. We must **rewire** how our brain associates movement—shifting it from a "chore" to something we **crave**.

> *"In the midst of movement and chaos, keep stillness inside of you."*
> —Deepak Chopra

Pain vs. Pleasure: Rewiring the Mind for Moving Meditation

One of the most powerful tools for habit change is understanding how your brain associates **pain** and **pleasure** with behaviors. If something feels painful, you avoid it. If it brings pleasure, you crave it. But what if your brain has been trained to seek pleasure in the wrong places (like numbing out with substances or unhealthy distractions) while seeing the things that actually help (like meditation or movement) as effort or obligation?

This is where **Neuro-Associative Conditioning (NAC)**—as taught by Tony Robbins in his book *Awaken the Giant Within*, and the habit formation principles in James Clear's *Atomic Habits*—come into play. The goal is to **reprogram your subconscious associations** so that Moving Meditation becomes something you instinctively seek out because it feels good, while staying stagnant feels like being stuck in a cage.

Step 1: Associate Pain with Inaction

If you continue avoiding movement, what are the consequences? What pain does inaction bring to your life? Think about:

- The **stress and anxiety** that build up when your mind races and you have no healthy way to release it

- Feeling **stuck in repetitive thought loops** because you never engage the body to help break the cycle

- The **physical tension** and **discomfort** that accumulate from inactivity, leading to stiffness, headaches, and fatigue

- The **frustration** and **guilt** of knowing that you need a solution but not taking action

Step 2: Link Massive Pleasure to Moving Meditation

Now, contrast that image with the incredible benefits of Moving Meditation. Imagine yourself embracing movement daily and how it changes everything:

- Your **mind feels clear**, your body energized, and your breath deep and steady.

- Instead of battling thoughts, you **channel them into fluid motion**, feeling present and free.

- Movement **washes away stress**, like stepping into a flowing river that clears mental clutter.

- Your body feels **stronger, more flexible, and resilient**, and you wake up each day with a sense of vitality.

- You gain a **natural dopamine boost**, replacing artificial highs with sustainable well-being.

Step 3: Reinforce the New Association Daily

To make this shift permanent, you must **remind yourself consistently** of the pain of inaction and the pleasure of movement. Try the following:

- Every morning, before you move, recall the pain of staying stuck. Then **visualize the pleasure of moving**.

- Create an affirmation or include in your Personal Power Affirmation: **"I embrace movement as a source of strength, resilience, and joy. Every step I take energizes my body and clears my mind."**

- When resistance shows up, ask yourself: **"Do I want to feel trapped and restless, or do I want to feel light and free?"**

- **Celebrate each session**, no matter how small. Your brain strengthens pleasurable habits when rewarded.

- **Pair Moving Meditation with a small joy**—your favorite playlist, stretching in the sun, or the peaceful silence of early morning.

The more you consciously associate **pleasure with movement** and **pain with inaction**, the more your brain will naturally pull you toward the right choice. Eventually, Moving Meditation won't be something you "have to" do—it'll be something you **actively seek out**.

Momhak Moment: Breaking a Craving Through Motion

One evening, that familiar tension crept in—the kind that used to push me toward drinking. The urge was there, buzzing in the background, tempting me to numb out. Instead of giving in, I stood up, walked outside, and started moving.
A slow stretch, a deep inhale, a few deliberate steps. Within minutes, something shifted. The craving lost its grip. My mind wasn't circling around it anymore—it was following my body's rhythm. By the time I got back inside, I didn't need a drink. I'd already found my release.

Foundations of Yoga, Tai Chi, Qi Gong & Moving Meditation

Moving Meditation can take many forms, but three of the most beginner-friendly approaches are **yoga, Tai Chi,** and **Qi Gong**. Each has distinct characteristics, yet all share core principles: **mindful movement, breath awareness,** and **inner focus**.

Remember, nearly any physical activity can become a form of Moving Meditation when you slow your pace, sync your breath with movement, and stay mindfully aware of your body's sensations, posture, and flow.

My Moving Meditation Routine

Over the years, I've refined my personal practice into a fluid, intentional sequence that blends Qi Gong, Tai Chi, and yoga into a deeply restorative and energizing Moving Meditation. Each session is a journey through breath, movement, and mindfulness, designed to awaken the body, calm the mind, and cultivate balance while building strength and flexibility.

- I begin with **Qi Gong**, using it as a warm-up to gently awaken my energy. The slow, rhythmic movements synchronize with my breath, helping me ground myself and clear any residual tension before transitioning into the next phase.

- From there, I move into a **short-form Yang-style Tai Chi** sequence. This practice emphasizes smooth, deliberate transitions, reinforcing relaxation and internal focus while improving strength and coordination. The meditative flow of Tai Chi brings me fully into the present moment, sharpening my awareness of each step and breath.

- Once my body is open and aligned, I transition into **three variations of sun salutations**—one that emphasizes lower body strength and flexibility, another that targets the upper body, and a third that engages the entire body for a balanced blend of strength and mobility. These dynamic sequences elevate my heart rate, build warmth, and engage my entire body.

- To conclude, I transition into a **yin yoga stretch session**, allowing my muscles to fully release and integrate the benefits of the practice. Holding postures for extended

101

periods encourages deep relaxation and targets the fascia, promoting flexibility and a profound sense of stillness.

This routine is more than just a physical exercise—it's a Moving Meditation, a way to align my breath, body, and mind in perfect harmony. It sets the tone for my day, leaving me feeling balanced, resilient, and connected.

Yoga: Linking Breath, Strength & Flexibility

As I'm sure you're aware, yoga is an ancient practice that integrates **movement, breath control,** and **mindfulness**. Rooted in India, it merges **physical postures (asanas)** with **breath control (pranayama)** and a mental framework for well-being.

Why Yoga Helps Recovery

Regulates the Nervous System: Reduces stress and anxiety

Improves Flexibility & Posture: Loosens tight muscles, promotes alignment

Builds Strength & Endurance: Strengthens muscles, improves balance

Encourages Self-Awareness: Keeps you present in your body

Simple Yoga Practices for Moving Meditation

Sun Salutations: A flowing sequence linking breath to each pose

Yin Yoga: Long-held stretches for deeper tissue release and relaxation

Restorative Yoga: Gentle, supportive postures for maximum relaxation

Try This: **A 5-minute yin yoga stretch to start your day**. Breathe deeply, move slowly, and focus on every sensation.

To deepen your yoga practice, consider exploring different styles and teachers. Attending a class, following guided online sessions, or working with an instructor can help refine your technique and understanding. There are countless resources available, from structured courses to free videos. For additional guidance and demonstrations, visit **Momhak.com**.

Tai Chi: Meditation in Motion

An ancient Chinese martial art, Tai Chi is often dubbed "meditation in motion" because its slow, graceful moves demand constant mindfulness.

Why Tai Chi Helps Recovery

Mind-Body Coordination: Requires focus on balance and fluid transitions

Relaxation & Craving Reduction: Calms the nervous system, diminishing triggers (Wayne & Fuerst, 2013)

Building Patience & Resilience: Fosters gentle self-regulation

Deep Breathing: Each movement paired with the breath, activating the parasympathetic system

Simple Tai Chi Practices

Short Forms (5 to 10 min): Basic, slow-flowing routines

Slow Weight Shifting: Inhale as you shift weight to one foot, then exhale as you return

Tai Chi Walk: An ultra-slow walk, each step measured and synced with your breath

Tai Chi Walk: Cultivating Balance and Mindfulness Through Movement

The **Tai Chi Walk** is a foundational practice in Tai Chi that emphasizes **slow, controlled steps** synchronized with **deep, Mindful Breathing**. It improves **balance, focus,** and **relaxation** while strengthening the connection between breath and movement. Unlike ordinary walking, the Tai Chi Walk requires **intentional**

shifting of weight, fluid motion, and heightened awareness of each step.

How to Perform the Tai Chi Walk

1. Start in a Relaxed, Centered Position

- Stand with feet hip to shoulder-width apart, knees slightly bent
- Keep your spine straight, shoulders relaxed, and gaze forward
- Place your hands gently at your sides

2. Shift Your Weight, Then Step Forward

- Slowly shift your weight onto your right foot as you inhale deeply through the nose
- Lift your left foot just off the ground, keeping it relaxed
- Extend the left foot forward and place the heel down first while keeping most of your weight on the back leg

3. Transfer Weight Gradually

- As you exhale slowly through the mouth, begin shifting your weight forward onto the left foot
- Feel the smooth transition as your back foot becomes lighter
- Once fully balanced on the left foot, lift the right foot off the ground for the next step

4. Repeat the Process

- Continue moving forward at a slow, controlled pace, fully shifting weight before lifting the back foot
- Maintain deep, rhythmic breathing—inhale as you lift and step, exhale as you shift and root
- Stay relaxed, keeping movements fluid, soft, and intentional

5. Maintain Awareness

- Focus on each movement, each breath, and each point of contact with the ground

- Imagine gliding forward smoothly, as if moving through water

- Keep your mind calm and present, fully engaged in the act of walking

One Mindful Step Right Now: If possible, stand up and take just **one** step forward as mindfully as possible. Feel your weight shift, your foot lift, moving through the air, and connecting with the ground. Take one step back in the same way. What did you notice in that single, focused movement?

How to Learn Tai Chi

The best way to experience Tai Chi is through consistent practice. Whether joining a local class, following online tutorials, or simply dedicating a few minutes each day to practice the Tai Chi Walk, you'll notice its calming effects over time. There are many great teachers and resources available online. Visit **Momhak.com** for videos and further insights into incorporating Tai Chi into your recovery journey.

Qi Gong: Cultivating Life-Force Energy

Qi Gong, a practice rooted in Traditional Chinese Medicine, focuses on cultivating Qi (life force energy) through a combination of movement, breathwork, and visualization. Some forms of Qi Gong emphasize physical movement, others integrate both movement and mental imagery, and some rely entirely on visualization alone, guiding energy flow purely through focused intention and breath awareness.

Scientifically, Qi can be described as a **bioelectromagnetic energy** that influences physiological processes in the body. Research in **biophysics** and **Traditional Chinese Medicine** suggests that Qi may correspond to **measurable electromagnetic fields** generated by the nervous system and cellular activity. Studies on **bioelectric**

fields, fascia conductivity, and **microcirculation** propose that Qi may relate to:

- **Bioelectric Signals** – Electrical impulses generated by the nervous system and muscles

- **Biomagnetic Fields** – Measurable magnetic fields produced by the heart and brain, which may influence cellular communication

- **Fascia as a Conductor** – The connective tissue network in the body, which some researchers suggest could facilitate the transmission of bioelectric energy

While modern science hasn't fully defined Qi in Western biomedical terms, **the existence of bioelectromagnetic fields in the body aligns with Qi's described role in Traditional Chinese Medicine** as an energetic force that supports circulation, healing, and overall balance.

Why Qi Gong Works for Recovery

Energy Flow: Balances and revitalizes the body's Qi (Chen et al., 2019)

Stress & Emotional Release: Clears blocked energy that can fuel anxiety or cravings

Enhanced Focus: The synergy of breath and movement grounds the mind

The Power of Visualization: Engaging the mind in guided imagery enhances the effects of Qi Gong, reinforcing the body's ability to self-regulate, reduce pain perception, and improve emotional resilience. Studies suggest that visualization can activate similar neural pathways as physical movement, helping to strengthen the mind-body connection even when stillness is practiced (Liu et al., 2023)

Simple Qi Gong Practices

Microcosmic Orbit: Circulate breath-energy up the spine (inhale) and down the front (exhale)

Gathering Qi: Raise and lower arms in tandem with inhales and exhales

Cloud Hands: Slow, sweeping movements to promote ease and presence

Exercise: Microcosmic Orbit Flow with Arm Movements

This exercise combines **breathwork, visualization,** and **flowing arm movements** to enhance relaxation and energy circulation through the body.

How to Practice:

1. Start in a Standing Position

- Stand with feet hip-width apart, knees slightly bent, back strait, and chin tucked.

- Relax your shoulders and do a few rounds of abdominal/diaphragmatic breathing, paying more attention to the exhalations than the inhalations. Gently press the tip of your tongue on the palate of your mouth.

2. Inhale – Arms Rise – Energy Moves Up the Spine

- As you **inhale**, raise your arms slowly up your sides, keeping them straight, palms facing down, and fingers together.

- Imagine energy rising from the base of the spine (Huiyin point) up along your **back to the crown of your head**.

- Keep the move smooth and continuous, ending with your arms lifted to shoulder or head height.

3. Exhale – Arms Lower – Energy Moves Down the Front Centerline

- As your inhale peaks, begin your exhale and bring your hands together in front of your face, palms facing inward.

- Continue the **exhale slowly** as your **hands move down the front of your body**, tracing a path from your face to your lower abdomen.

- Visualize energy flowing **down the front of your body**, from the crown of your head to just below the navel.

4. Repeat & Flow

- Continue this movement for **5 to 10 minutes**, synchronizing your breath with your movement.

- Feel the energy moving smoothly in a continuous circle **up the back, over the head, down the front**, and **through the legs**.

5. Complete the Cycle – Return to Center

- To end the exercise, bring your hands gently to rest over your lower abdomen, one hand placed on top of the other. Let your palms softly cradle your belly, with your thumbs touching, forming a small hollow where your belly button sits nestled between them. This position helps you anchor attention in your body's energetic center, which is located just below the navel.

- Take a few rounds of slow, diaphragmatic breathing, allowing your abdomen to rise and fall naturally beneath your hands. With each breath, feel your energy gathering and consolidating in your core.

- This is your return point—your center. End your practice with calm awareness and gratitude for the energy you've cultivated.

- To finish, rub your hands briskly together then massage your face, head, ears, and neck.

How to Learn Qi Gong

Qi Gong is best learned through direct experience. Whether practicing with an instructor, following online sessions, or integrating simple movements into your daily routine, regular practice will help you tap into its full benefits. There are many excellent videos and teachers available online. For further guidance, visit **Momhak.com**.

Movement as a Shield Against Stress

I used to buckle under stress and anxiety. When something triggered me, I'd feel it in my chest—a tightness, a shortness of breath. My default reaction was to escape, to numb it. But one day, instead of reaching for a distraction, I stepped onto my mat and went through a simple sun salutation routine. It took all of 5 minutes, but by the end, the tension had melted—not through avoidance but through presence. It was a simple shift but a profound one: I'd replaced my escape route with a reset button—and it was built into my own breath and body.

The Hidden Power of Spinal Movement

When you observe masters of Tai Chi, Yoga, or Qi Gong, you might notice their fluid grace—but beneath that visible elegance lies a critical element: **intentional spinal movement**. While modern life relegates our spine to a rigid pole (hunched over devices or locked in office chairs), these ancient practices recognize the spine as the body's central communication highway.

Spinal Fluidity: The Missing Link

The spine houses your nervous system—the very network transmitting signals between brain and body. When we maintain spinal mobility through gentle, deliberate movement, we:

- Enhance neural communication between brain and body

- Regulate the autonomic nervous system, shifting from stress to calm

- Release tension that often triggers emotional reactivity

- Improve circulation to brain and vital organs

This helps explain why, after a Tai Chi session or yoga flow, your mind feels sharper and emotions more balanced. This is because you've literally improved the physical conduit of your thoughts and feelings.

How Ancient Practices Activate the Spine

Each tradition approaches spinal movement differently:

- **Yoga** systematically moves through spinal planes with forward folds, backbends, twists, and lateral stretches, releasing trapped energy described as "prana."

- **Tai Chi** emphasizes the subtle "wave" through the spine during transitions, teaching practitioners to initiate movement from the center and let it ripple outward.

- **Qi Gong** focuses on gentle spinal rotations and undulations that help energy (qi) flow through meridians, many of which run parallel to the spine.

Science Corner: Spinal Movement & Stress Relief

A systematic review and meta-analysis published in the *Journal of Clinical Medicine* found that mind-body exercises significantly improved heart rate variability parameters and reduced perceived stress levels (Zou et al., 2018). These movements, which prominently feature controlled spinal motion, appear to directly influence autonomic nervous system function. Additional research shows increased activity in the prefrontal cortex—the area responsible for executive function and emotional control—following movement practices that engage the full spine.

Simple Spinal Integration

Even if you can't commit to a full yoga or Tai Chi class, you can incorporate spinal movement into daily life with the following methods:

Morning Awakening: While still in bed, lift your knees and gently roll them side to side while keeping your shoulders flat on the bed.

Desk Breaks: Every hour, perform a gentle seated twist, looking over each shoulder while keeping your hips forward.

Walking Meditation: Consciously allow your spine to move naturally as you walk rather than holding it rigidly.

Momhak Moment

Your spine isn't just structural support—it's the bridge between mind and body. Each gentle twist, bend, or rotation recalibrates this connection, bringing you back to center.

Mind-Body Synergy

Moving Meditation doesn't just affect your **mental state**—it also has **direct physical benefits**:

- **Improved Flexibility & Posture** – Yoga and Tai Chi correct alignment and develop balance

- **Reduced Tension & Pain** – Lowers cortisol levels, easing stress-related aches

- **Enhanced Circulation & Organ Health** – Movement stimulates blood flow, lymphatic drainage, and oxygenation

Emotional Regulation & Stress Relief

Eckhart Tolle emphasizes that most human suffering comes from **non-acceptance of the present moment**. Moving Meditation interrupts this cycle by **rooting you in the now**.

Try This: Next time you sense stress building, respond with mindful motion—a slow step or a gentle stretch—letting the body guide you back to calm.

Integrating Affirmations & Breath

Pairing affirmations with movement reinforces positive mental shifts, as in the following exercise:

Choose a simple affirmation:

"I release stress" (inhale); "I embrace calm" (exhale).

"I am strong" (inhale); "I am resilient" (exhale).

Repeat during slow movement, allowing your body to absorb the message.

Try this: Walk slowly, synchronizing steps with your breath and silently affirming:

I move forward with ease. I am present, steady, and calm.

Tailoring Your Practice

Not everyone has an hour for mindful movement daily—and that's okay. **Short, consistent sessions** can also be incredibly transformative.

5-Minute Micro-Practices

Qi Gong: Arm raises while inhaling deeply for 2 or 3 minutes

Tai Chi: Tai Chi Walk or a simple short form

Yoga: A simple sun salutation routine

Try This: Stand, inhale, and raise your arms overhead for 4 seconds, then exhale while lowering your arms for 6 seconds. Just two minutes of this can reboot your mind.

Case Study: Anne (Early Recovery from Alcohol)

Anne, a 34-year-old nurse, needed an outlet for her mounting stress. She'd tried seated meditation but found her mind racing. Eventually, she discovered **flow yoga**. Starting with 10-minute morning sessions, she synced slow movements with deep inhales and exhales. Within weeks, she noticed:

• Reduced impulsive urges to drink after work

• Improved lower-back comfort from daily standing

• A calmer transition into bedtime

For Anne, **physical engagement** was the missing link. Instead of dreading "exercise," yoga became her morning relaxation time.

Overcoming Common Hurdles

"I don't have time."

Stack short sessions onto routine tasks, such as 5 minutes of Qi Gong while waiting for coffee to brew.

"I feel self-conscious."

Start at home or a private area. Confidence grows over time.

"I get impatient."

Set a 2-minute timer. Even 120 seconds of slow movement can break negative loops.

"It feels too slow."

Reframe "slow" as "intentional." The calm pace of movement is exactly what soothes restlessness.

Emergency 2-Minute Stress Craving Intervention

When cravings or stress strike, try this **movement-based sequence** in under 2 minutes. Craft an affirmation made of two lines: one that fits the rhythm of a 4-second inhale, and one that fits the rhythm of a 6-second exhale. Let the words match your breath. Stand or sit with your feet firmly grounded, and let your arms hang relaxed at your sides. Begin a simple flowing movement:

1. Inhale slowly for 4 seconds as you slowly lift your arms up in front of you, palms facing forward and fingers pointing inward while you repeat your 4-second affirmation.

2. Exhale slowly for 6 seconds as you lower your arms down in a circular motion along your sides, palms facing outward and fingers pointing up while you repeat your 6-second affirmation.

Repeat this breath-movement-affirmation cycle 6 times, letting your motion follow the rhythm of your breath.

Final Shift: Walk in place or do a gentle stretch for 30 seconds, bridging mind and body so that stress can't take hold.

#Momhak365 Challenge

Try this **2-minute intervention** whenever stress or cravings arise for a week. Jot down how you feel before and after, noticing how quickly movement replaces old coping mechanisms with genuine relief.

The Science of Flow: Why Movement Shifts Brain Chemistry

Psychologist Mihaly Csikszentmihalyi coined the term **"flow state"** to describe an immersive condition in which we become so engaged in an activity that **self-consciousness dissolves and time seems to disappear** (Csikszentmihalyi, 1990). This state is often described as a perfect balance between challenge and skill, where effort feels effortless and deep focus replaces external distractions. Many physical activities—like **Yoga, Tai Chi, Qi Gong,** and **mindful walking—can induce flow** because they **require a present-moment focus** and a synchronization of breath, movement, and awareness. These practices help bridge the **mind-body connection**, enhancing both cognitive function and emotional stability.

- **Challenge:** Staying present with each movement, adjusting postures, and refining balance

- **Skill:** Learning sequences progressively so that the movement remains engaging but not overwhelming

Neurochemical Effects of Flow

Entering a flow state triggers a cascade of neurochemical changes in the brain:

- **Dopamine Surge – Flow boosts dopamine,** a neurotransmitter linked to motivation, pleasure, and reward. This helps **reinforce positive behaviors** and strengthens neural pathways associated with learning and self-discipline.

114

- **Lowered Stress Hormones** – Cortisol (the primary stress hormone) drops significantly when we're in flow, **helping the nervous system shift from fight-or-flight mode to a more balanced state.** This is crucial for recovery from addiction, as stress resilience plays a key role in relapse prevention.

- **Increased Endorphins & Anandamide** – These natural mood enhancers reduce pain perception and promote feelings of relaxation and joy. This is why many people feel a deep sense of contentment after mindful movement practices.

Flow & Recovery: A Natural High

For those in recovery, achieving flow through Moving Meditation offers a **natural "high"** that **mimics the euphoria of addictive substances**—without the crash or negative consequences. Instead of seeking external rewards (like alcohol, drugs, or compulsive behaviors), the **brain rewires itself** to find pleasure and fulfillment in present-moment engagement. Over time, this shift **restores healthy dopamine balance**, making sobriety feel less like deprivation and more like an active, fulfilling state of being.

By engaging in intentional movement, breathwork, and meditative focus, we cultivate a sustainable source of pleasure, clarity, and emotional regulation—one that **supports long-term transformation** without reliance on artificial highs.

The Weekly Moving Meditation Plan

Below is a sample schedule to help you integrate mindful movement into your daily life:

Day	Morning (5 to 10 mins)	Evening (5 to 15 mins)	Focus/Notes
Monday	Qi Gong	Yoga: Yin or restorative poses	Start gently; ease into the week

Tuesday	Mindful Walk (5–10 mins)	Tai Chi Walk	Replace anxious thoughts with physical flow
Wednesday	Yoga: Sun Salutations	Light stretch + 4–6 breathing	Observe mental chatter; use slow exhales
Thursday	Qi Gong	Tai Chi Walk	Compare energy levels a.m. vs. p.m.
Friday	Yoga: Sun Salutations	Yoga: Yin or restorative poses	End the week in relaxed presence
Saturday	Your choice	Your choice	Explore variety; see what resonates most
Sunday	Gentle walk + breathwork	Rest day or small stretch	Reflect on changes in mood, cravings, and energy

Reflection: Each night, note any shifts in stress, cravings, or mood. Over time, notice which practices benefit you most.

Chapter 5 Summary: Moving Meditation

Core Message

Meditation isn't just about sitting still. Movement—through yoga, Tai Chi, Qi Gong, or nearly any physical activity done mindfully—can transform your brain, reduce stress, and ease your recovery.

Key Lessons

Movement can be meditation: You don't have to sit quietly—rhythmic, mindful motion grounds the mind in the present.

Let breath guide your motion: Inhale as you stretch upward, and exhale as you sink lower into the movement. Rather than forcing breath control, let your body naturally sync with the rhythm—step, inhale, shift, exhale. The movement itself becomes the meditation

Small, consistent practice leads to long-term transformation. Even 5 minutes a day can reset how you handle stress and cravings.

Quick Win for Today: 2-Minute Moving Meditation

1. Stand comfortably with your eyes closed.

2. Inhale (4 seconds) raising your arms, then exhale (6 seconds) lowering them.

3. Repeat for 2 minutes, focusing on breath and motion.

4. Do you feel calmer, more centered?

You've just performed a Moving Meditation. Even small moments of presence can rewire your stress response.

Your #Momhak365 Challenge: 5 Minutes Daily

For the next **7 days**, dedicate **5 minutes** to mindful movement:

- **Tai Chi**: Tai Chi Walk or a simple short form
- **Yoga**: A few slow, deliberate postures
- **Qi Gong**: Arm-raising flows or Cloud Hands
- **Mindful Walk**: Breathe in sync with each step

Track: How you feel before and after. Over time, notice:

- Emotional stability and lower stress
- Enhanced body awareness and control
- A gentle dopamine lift from physical engagement

Bonus: Share your daily practice with **#Momhak365**, and join a community seeking the same transformation.

Looking Ahead: Mind Hacking & Thought Rewiring

In Chapter 6, we'll explore the power of **mind hacking**, which involves:

- Reprogramming negative loops and destructive mental habits

- Further exploring the Pain-Pleasure Principle

- Examining why affirmations and cognitive reframing truly work

Your **mind** follows your **movement**—now let's reprogram it.

CHAPTER 6: MIND HACKING - REWIRE YOUR THOUGHTS & RECLAIM YOUR LIFE

WHAT YOU'LL DISCOVER

- How to rewire negative thought patterns and break destructive mental loops
- The power of affirmations, reframing, and cognitive-behavioral techniques
- How to use the Pain-Pleasure Principle to reprogram cravings
- Why self-forgiveness is key to lasting transformation

KEY INSIGHTS

- Your thoughts shape your reality—changing them changes everything
- Reframing automatic negative thoughts weakens addiction's hold
- The pleasure–pain principle (Tony Robbins' Neuro-Associative Conditioning) makes sobriety more rewarding
- Self-forgiveness releases guilt and allows real healing to begin

YOUR TRANSFORMATION TOOLS

- Cognitive Reframing – Catch, challenge, and replace negative thoughts
- Pleasure–Pain Reset – Associate massive pain with the addiction; associate pleasure with freedom

- Affirmations – Rewire beliefs through repetition and embodiment

- Forgiveness Practice – Techniques to release guilt and break free from self-blame

"We are what we repeatedly do. Excellence, then, is not an act, but a habit."
—Aristotle

Mind Hacking for Real Change

Up to now, you've learned how Cold Exposure, Mindful Breathing, and Moving Meditation can reset your body and calm your mind. In this chapter, we'll dig deeper into the mental realm—the thoughts, beliefs, and emotional patterns that've guided your behavior, often without your conscious awareness. By "hacking" these internal patterns, you'll gain the power to disrupt addictive cycles, rewire your mindset, and anchor yourself in a new, positive identity.

Mind Hacking is the process of intentionally dismantling these harmful cycles and replacing them with patterns that nurture growth. In doing so, you gain the power to choose responses overreacting on autopilot. This shift is profound because it stops addictive urges at their source: the stories playing out in your mind, often without your conscious consent.

Below, you'll discover practical techniques ranging from affirmations to cognitive reframing (a bedrock of modern psychology) and Tony Robbins' Neuro-Associative Conditioning, plus the art of self-forgiveness. Each method helps you rewrite the scripts that drive destructive behaviors, empowering you to anchor in a healthy, creative, and free version of yourself.

"It's the repetition of affirmations that leads to belief. And once that belief becomes a deep conviction, things begin to happen."
—Muhammad Ali

Affirmations

Before we dive into specific affirmation techniques, it's important to understand why these aren't just empty words or wishful thinking. Affirmations are powerful neural tools that literally reshape how your brain processes information about yourself and your abilities. They can:

1. **Activate Reward Centers:** Neuroimaging shows increased activity in motivation-related areas when using affirmations—the same regions that help drive positive behavior and strengthen resilience.

2. **Buffer Stress:** Affirmations help maintain performance under pressure. When you're facing cravings or triggers, these mental anchors can keep you steady.

3. **Enhance Motivation:** Repeating desired traits or outcomes strengthens neural circuits that drive those behaviors. Think of it as building mental muscle memory for the mindset you want to embody.

The power of affirmations lies in their ability to speak directly to your subconscious mind. While your conscious mind may resist change ("I've tried to quit before and failed"), affirmations bypass this resistance by planting seeds of possibility that grow stronger with repetition.

I often pair affirmations with my breath holds during Tummo/Wim Hof breathing exercises. There's something powerful about linking a **physical challenge** (holding my breath) with a **mental statement** ("I'm relaxed, confident and content, thriving in complete sobriety"). This layered approach creates a sense of clarity and conviction that pure words alone can't match.

Creating Effective Affirmations

To genuinely rewire your brain, affirmations should be:

1. Realistic: Sticking to language that you can believe

2. Positive, Not Negative: "I am strong!"

3. Present-Tense: "I am" rather than "I will be"

4. Personally Meaningful & Connected with Core Values: Reflect your unique goals and challenges

5. Emotional: Recite them with feeling, not just by rote

6. Consistent: The neural pathways form through repetition over time

When to Practice:

- **Just before sleeping** (your mind continues to process these thoughts as you're asleep)

- **Upon waking** (to set a positive tone for the day)

- **When looking in the mirror**

- **During Mindful Breathing or Cold Exposure** (heightened focus can deepen affirmations)

- **Whenever stress or cravings appear** (affirmations serve as a mental "pause button")

Weaving Affirmations Throughout

Don't limit affirmations to morning or bedtime—experiment with sprinkling them throughout the day. Use them before a meeting, while walking, during stress, or on your way to a social function. Affirmations become your mental shield against old neural loops.

Visualization & Affirmations

Don't just say the words—**see** them. Picture yourself thriving in everyday life: feeling energetic at sunrise, enjoying genuine conversations, and accomplishing goals. Engage all your senses to make these scenarios as real as possible. The brain learns best from vivid, emotional experiences.

Practical Tip: Combine visualization with music that inspires you or triggers a sense of calm. This multisensory approach can amplify the emotional impact of your affirmations, further anchoring them in your neural pathways.

"I would visualize things coming to me. It would just make me feel better. Visualization works if you work hard. That's the thing. You can't just visualize and go eat a sandwich."
—Jim Carrey

Science Corner: Why Layered Mind Practices Work

Your brain doesn't change through willpower alone—it changes through consistent, reinforced experience. Cognitive reprogramming works best when it's supported on multiple fronts. Think of the Four Pillars not as isolated hacks but as synchronized signals that strengthen the same message: **You are changing**. When you pair affirmations with deep breathwork, or repeat empowering beliefs while taking a cold shower, you're not just "being positive"—you're forging stronger, more resilient neural networks. Research in neuroplasticity shows that when multiple senses and systems are engaged at once, the brain encodes the experience more deeply. In simple terms: **the more immersive the change, the more permanent it becomes.**

This is one of the hidden strengths of The Momhak Method. By combining techniques—like cognitive reframing with embodied practices—you multiply their effect. You're not trying to **force** your brain into a new state—you're creating a web of reinforcing inputs that make the new way feel natural. Just as a tree is more stable when its roots grow in multiple directions, your new mindset holds stronger when it's anchored through multiple daily practices.

The Tony Robbins Spin on Affirmations

Renowned life coach Tony Robbins used to jog while repeating statements like "I am unstoppable!" at full volume. Pairing affirmations with movement floods your brain with endorphins, tying positive language to physical momentum. This technique speeds up the **rewiring** of self-belief into your nervous system.

NAC: Neuro-Associative Conditioning

Tony Robbins' **Neuro-Associative Conditioning (NAC)** is built on a fundamental truth about human motivation: **we always do more to avoid pain than to seek pleasure**. This principle is especially powerful when it comes to breaking addictive habits. By rewiring the brain's associations, you can disrupt destructive patterns and create a compelling future that naturally pulls you forward.

Instead of relying on willpower alone, NAC reprograms your brain by linking **massive pain** to an old habit while amplifying the **pleasure of transformation**. This shift engages your emotions at the deepest level, making change not just desirable—it makes it *inevitable*.

Step 1: Identify the Habit You Want to Change

Write down the exact behavior that holds you back. Be brutally honest, as in these examples:

- "I drink alcohol when I'm stressed."

- "I binge on junk food when I feel lonely."

- "I waste hours scrolling on my phone instead of doing meaningful activities."

Naming the habit brings clarity, which is the first step toward breaking free.

Step 2: Associate Massive Pain with the Old Habit

Your brain avoids what it perceives as painful. If you haven't changed a habit yet, it's because the pain of quitting doesn't outweigh the pain of continuing. It's time to flip that balance.

Exercise: List every negative consequence of your habit. Dig deep and **feel** the weight of these consequences.

- **Financial loss:** How much money has this habit cost you?

- **Health deterioration:** How has it impacted your body, energy, and longevity?

- **Broken relationships:** Has it distanced you from loved ones?

- **Mental toll:** Does it make you feel trapped, ashamed, or stuck in a cycle?

- **Lost opportunities:** What have you missed out on because of this habit?

- **Loss of self-respect:** How does it make you feel about yourself?

Let this list sink in, and imagine experiencing these pains at their worst. The goal is to make your current habit feel unbearable.

Step 3: Load the Pleasure of Change

Once you've anchored enough pain to the old habit, shift gears. The brain needs a compelling alternative to move toward.

Exercise: Visualize your best self, completely free from this habit. Write down every benefit of this change, such as:

- **Physical well-being:** Waking up energized, strong, and clear-headed

- **Emotional stability:** Confidence, self-respect, and emotional resilience

- **Stronger relationships:** More meaningful connections with friends and family

- **Financial gain:** Saving money and investing in experiences that bring true fulfillment

- **Inner peace:** A sense of calm, knowing that you're in control.

Close your eyes and **immerse yourself in this future**. Picture yourself living in this reality. What does it feel like? The more vividly you can experience this shift, the more compelling it becomes.

Step 4: Reinforce the Shift with Mental Reminders

To solidify the transformation, create daily mental cues that keep you anchored in your new reality.

Pain-Pleasure Journal: Keep a small notebook (or note on your phone) with two columns: **Pain of the Old Habit** and **Pleasure of the New Life**. Read this list every morning and whenever cravings strike.

Vision Board: Assemble images that represent your best self—fit, confident, and thriving in meaningful activities. Let these visuals remind you of what's at stake.

Daily Affirmations: Pair your new identity with powerful self-talk: "I am strong, free, and in control."

Essential for Early Recovery

In the beginning stages of sobriety, it's essential to pair **positive affirmations** with a clear acknowledgment of alcohol's negative impact.

Take 2 minutes daily to reinforce this shift:

1. **Recall the pain and consequences** your bad habit has caused—physically, mentally, and emotionally.

2. **Shift into uplifting, forward-focused affirmations,** reminding yourself of the rewards of a sober, healthy life.

Why This Works: The brain responds powerfully to contrast. Acknowledging past pain clarifies your "Why", while affirmations reprogram your focus toward progress. Over time, this conditioning rewires cravings, making sobriety feel not like deprivation but liberation instead.

Final Takeaway: Make Sobriety More Rewarding Than the Old Habit

Breaking free from addiction isn't about just avoiding alcohol or another habit—it's also about **building a life that feels so rich and fulfilling that relapse isn't even tempting**.

- Associate **massive pain** with the old pattern

- Attach **intense pleasure** to your transformation

- Use **daily reinforcement tools** to lock in these new beliefs

Cognitive Behavioral Therapy (CBT): The Gold Standard

While NAC leans heavily on motivational imagery, **cognitive behavioral therapy (CBT)** offers a more clinical, research-backed approach to treating addictions, anxiety, and depression. As outlined in the 1994 book *Cognitive Therapy of Substance Abuse* (Beck, Wright, Newman, and Liese), CBT focuses on identifying and correcting "automatic negative thoughts" that fuel addictive behaviors and provides a structured way to catch and replace them.

1. Recognize Automatic Thoughts

You might think, *I'm weak—I can't handle stress without a drink* without even realizing it.

2. Challenge Them

- Is this thought really true?

- What evidence do you have?

- Has it always happened every time?

- Are there moments you succeeded that you're ignoring?

3. Replace

- *I've made progress before, and I can do it again.*

- *I'm learning better strategies every day.*

Quick Hack to Interrupt Negative Loops

Let's start with a **30-second mind hack** that can instantly shift you from self-doubt to determination. This is your "grab-and-go" strategy, ideal for moments when cravings spike or self-criticism runs wild.

1. Spot a Negative Thought

- Notice one self-defeating idea, like *I'll never stay sober around my old friends*

- Don't judge it, but instead recognize it as a passing leaf atop the river of your mind

2. Pause & Breathe

Close your eyes. Inhale for 4 seconds, exhale for 6.

3. Question Its Truth

- Ask: *Is this 100% accurate? Could I see this differently?*

- A negative thought is usually an exaggeration, not a law of reality

4. Insert an Empowering Alternative

- Example: *I'm learning and growing. Each step makes me stronger.*

- Speak it out loud if possible—the resonance of your voice helps encode new neural pathways

5. Visualize Success

Picture yourself acting on this new belief—refusing a drink at a gathering, taking a calming breath instead of lashing out, or choosing an affirmation over self-criticism.

The Thought Reframe Journal

Just like lifting weights builds muscle, training your brain to reframe thoughts builds resilience.

Keep this simple:

- **One Negative Thought You Noticed**
  Example: *I can't handle stress without alcohol.*

- **Reframe the Thought into an Empowering Truth**
  Example: *I'm learning to navigate stress with movement and breath.*

- **One Action You Took to Reinforce the New Thought**
  Example: *Took a 5-minute walk instead of drinking.*

Over 7 days, watch how reframing plus small actions can shift your entire mindset.

Writing down your reframes makes them tangible. Some people find an extra boost by sharing a particularly powerful affirmation or successful reframe, perhaps using **#Momhak365**. Witnessing each other's mental shifts reinforces that this rewiring process truly works.

Emotional Regulation: Name It to Tame It

Identify vs. Suppress

A critical piece of Mind Hacking is learning to face emotions honestly rather than numbing or running from them. People often drink or use substances to avoid discomfort—like anxiety, anger, or loneliness. But ignoring these feelings simply delays the pain (and often intensifies it).

Name It to Tame It: The next time you feel that tightness in your chest or jittery tension in your stomach, say out loud (or in your head): "I feel anxiety in my chest" or "I notice sadness in my throat."

Pause & Breathe: Take a 30-second pause to do a mini breathing reset of your choice, whether 4–6 or 4–7–8. Remind yourself that it's just a feeling—one that will pass if you allow it to.

Quick Script:

"I notice that I feel tense; let me pause and breathe. I am safe in this moment. This feeling will pass."

By naming your emotion, you "step outside" of it, reducing its intensity and making it less likely you'll default to harmful coping mechanisms.

Why This Matters

Breaking an addictive cycle requires emotional self-awareness. If you can recognize your stress or sadness early, you have a chance to respond with a healthy tool—like affirmations, a quick walk, or reaching out to a supportive friend—instead of reaching for a substance.

Even a 30-second mindfulness break can shift your emotional state. For instance, a study at the University of California indicated that labeling an emotion in real-time (such as "I feel anger") decreased physiological arousal, lowering both heart rate and cortisol levels (Lieberman et al. 2007). This is a deceptively simple yet potent strategy that can prevent relapse moments before it happens.

Self-Forgiveness: The Key to Releasing Shame & Moving Forward

Guilt can be a useful signal when it prompts you to correct a mistake. But prolonged guilt morphs into **shame**—the belief "I am bad" rather than the statement "I did something bad." Shame traps you in a cycle of self-loathing that ironically drives you back to the very substances or behaviors you're trying to escape.

The next time guilt arises, **use this 3-step process:**

1. Acknowledge the Regret (Without Judgment)

Ask yourself:

- *What am I feeling guilty about?*

- *How is this guilt serving me?*

Shift your mindset:

- **Instead of:** *I was selfish and hurt people.*

- **Think:** *I was struggling, and I didn't have the tools I have now. I choose to do better.*

Why This Works:

When people acknowledge their guilt with compassion rather than judgment, they're more likely to take positive action rather than relapse into self-destructive behavior.

2. Reframe the Mistake as a Lesson, Not a Life Sentence
Ask yourself:

- *If a friend made the same mistake, how would I support them?*

- *What did I learn from this experience that I can apply going forward?*

Example Reframe:

Instead of: *I let people down, and they'll never trust me again.*

Think: *I'm learning to rebuild trust through consistent actions.*

Why This Works:

The more you frame past mistakes as opportunities for growth, the less power they have over your present.

3. Release & Replace with an Empowering Thought
Final step:

- Close your eyes for a moment and imagine the weight of guilt lifting from your shoulders.

- Take a deep breath in, and as you exhale, let go of that past version of yourself.

Repeat this self-forgiveness affirmation:

I release the weight of my past. I am learning, growing, and moving forward.

Why This Works:

Replacing self-critical thoughts with empowering beliefs can significantly reduce stress and increase resilience in recovery.

Momhak Moment

Forgiving yourself isn't about excusing the harm that's been done—it's about breaking the chains of regret so that you can truly move forward.

Quick Win: Forgive Past Regrets

Write down a list of past regrets, then write a compassionate reframe for each one—turning guilt into growth by acknowledging what you learned and how you've changed.

Beyond the Victim Mindset

Victimhood vs. Empowerment

In her groundbreaking work at Stanford University's Addiction Medicine Clinic, Dr. Anna Lembke discovered something crucial—that the mindset we adopt about our struggles can either lock us in addiction or propel us toward freedom. Her research, documented in her 2021 book *Dopamine Nation,* reveals how victim mentality actually changes our brain's reward circuitry, making recovery more difficult.

Practical Steps to Shift Your Mindset

1. Identify Victim Language

Research from cognitive behavioral therapy shows that language shapes reality. Notice phrases like:

- *Why does this always happen to me?*

- *Nothing ever works out for me.*

- *I'm cursed/unlucky/doomed.*

2. Reframe Each Challenge

Reframing adversity as opportunity activates regions in the brain associated with resilience and growth. For each struggle, ask:

- *What can I learn from this?*

- *How might this make me stronger?*

132

- *What skills am I developing by facing this?*

3. Take Responsibility Without Shame

Dr. Lembke's clinical work shows that accepting responsibility while releasing shame is crucial for transformation. This means:

- Acknowledging your role in situations
- Focusing on what you can control
- Viewing past actions as learning experiences

Dr. Carol Dweck on Growth Mindset

In her 2006 book *Mindset: The New Psychology of Success*, Dweck notes that people who view challenges as opportunities for growth—rather than unfair burdens—demonstrate:

- Enhanced resilience to stress
- Greater life satisfaction
- More effective and sustained behavioral changes

"A pessimist sees the difficulty in every opportunity; an optimist sees the opportunity in every difficulty."
—Winston Churchill

Neuroplastic Reinforcement in Daily Life: Consistency is Key

You'll remember that **neuroplasticity** (introduced in Chapter 2) is the continuous rewiring of your brain in response to repeated thoughts and behaviors. You essentially become what you repeatedly do.

- **Every Negative Thought Reframed** → Nudges your brain away from craving loops

133

- **Every Successful Craving Resistance** → Builds confidence and resilience, fueling the next successful resistance
- **Every Positive Affirmation** → Strengthens the neural networks of self-belief

Think of your mind as a **forest of neural trails**: Each time you choose a healthier path, you're trampling down weeds and creating a clearer, more navigable trail. Over weeks and months, these new trails become your **default**.

Momhak Moment

Your struggles aren't punishments—they're invitations to grow stronger. Every challenge is raw material for transformation.

Habit Stacking: The Key to Effortless Change

As James Clear emphasizes in *Atomic Habits*, **habit stacking** links a new behavior to something you already do automatically—like drinking morning coffee or brushing your teeth. This takes advantage of your existing routine to anchor the new habit until it becomes second nature.

Consider these combos:

1. After Brushing Your Teeth (Morning)

- **30 seconds of affirmations**: "I thrive in sobriety. I handle stress with grace. I love feeling strong and clear-headed."
- **15-second mindful breath**: Inhale for 4, exhale for 6.

2. While Waiting for Coffee

- **Quick Visualization**: Picture your day unfolding smoothly, with calm responses to any triggers.
- **Option**: Read your pain-pleasure list.

3. End-of-Day Wind-Down

- **Light Stretching** or yoga for 5 minutes.

- **Repeat an affirmation** about self-forgiveness or gratitude for the day's progress.

4. Moments of Stress & Negative Thought Loops

- **Keep a sticky note** on your desk: "4-6 breathing + Reframe." Each time stress spikes, do exactly that.

- **State your new script aloud** or internally. Feel the sense of empowerment from tackling discomfort head-on.

Bringing It All Together: A Sample Mind-Hacking Day

Morning

- Wake up → Inhale for 4, exhale for 6 → Affirmation: "I am strong, calm, and ready to grow."

- Quick 30-second cold water rinse in the middle of your shower → Reinforce with a statement like, "This resilience fuels my day."

Midday

- Notice a creeping negative thought: "I can't handle the stress of this job."

- Reframe: "I learn skills daily to manage stress. I'm stronger each time I practice."

- Action Step: 5-minute walk outside or a 5 minute 4–7–8 breath cycle.

Afternoon Craving

- Automatic thought: "I need a beer after work to decompress."

- Pain-pleasure: Recall the consequences (hangovers, regret) and the joys of new coping methods (better mood, clearer mind).

- Affirmation: "Freedom from alcohol feels amazing; I celebrate each sober evening with pride and self-respect."

Evening

- 5-minute easy yoga stretch → Affirmation: "I release today's worries. I rest in calm and look forward to tomorrow."

- Self-Forgiveness prompt: Reflect on any slip-ups. "I learn from my day. I forgive mistakes and embrace growth."

Over time, layering these small "hacks" transforms your daily routine into a powerful framework that reprograms how you handle emotions, stress, and self-doubt.

Quick Recap & Strategic Takeaways

Mind Hacking = Intentional Reprogramming

You intervene on autopilot thoughts, replacing them with new neural patterns that support sobriety.

Emotional Awareness vs. Emotional Avoidance

Let emotions surface, name them, and handle them with breathwork or reframing instead of burying bad habits or avoidance behaviors.

Self-Forgiveness Liberates Energy

Holding onto guilt or shame saps motivation. Releasing self-blame frees you to invest in healthy habits.

Victim Mindset vs. Growth Mindset

If you believe you're doomed, that belief can become self-fulfilling. Instead, adopt a perspective of **active participation** in your recovery and see obstacles as catalysts for learning.

Neuroplastic Reinforcement

Each positive shift, no matter how small, physically reshapes your brain. **Consistency**—not perfection—fuels sustainable change.

Habit Stacking

Seamlessly integrate new habits into existing routines. This approach ensures minimal friction and maximum staying power.

Tony Robbins' NAC:
Associate massive **pain with your old behaviors** and **massive pleasure with your new, sober life**.

CBT: Cognitive Behavioral Therapy
Build on the NAC principle with a structured format for identifying, challenging, and replacing negative thoughts.

Affirmation + Visualization:
Flood your mind with *I can*, *I am*, and *I choose*. Over time, **your brain believes what you consistently tell it**.

"Any idea, plan or purpose may be placed in the mind through repetition of thought."
—Napoleon Hill

Quick Win: Craft a Pain-Pleasure Affirmation

1. **Select your habit:** For example, quitting alcohol or smoking, or even negative self-talk.

2. **Identify the pain:** Write 3 bullet points describing the pain this habit brings you. Example: "I lose money, I lose respect, and I hurt my body."

3. **Identify the pleasure:** Write 3 bullet points of the blessings you'll gain by stopping. Example: "I'll have more money, more energy, and more confidence."

4. **Formulate a One-Sentence Affirmation:** Combine both. For instance:

   "Alcohol poisons my health, relationships and happiness. Thriving in sobriety brings me real joy, calmness, and success."

5. **Say It Daily:** Morning, before bed, and whenever a craving strikes.

Chapter 6 Summary: Mind Hacking

Core Message

Your thoughts shape your reality. To break free from addiction, you must rewire limiting beliefs, reframe cravings, and program your brain for success. Mind Hacking means spotting disempowering beliefs and habits and systematically replacing them with convictions that align with health, resilience, and hope.

Key Lessons

Negative Thought Loops → These keep you stuck in addictive ruts. Identifying and reframing them is your golden ticket to freedom.

Tony Robbins' Pain–Pleasure Principle → Paint the old habit as deeply painful and the new lifestyle as invigorating—this realigns your motivation system.

CBT & Reframing → Deliberately reprogram automatic thoughts. Over time, your mind rewires to prefer sober, healthy coping strategies.

Self-Forgiveness → Guilt is a teacher, not a life sentence. Release shame, embrace growth.

Victim vs. Growth Mindset → See your struggles as stepping stones, not dead ends. Accepting personal power accelerates progress.

Neuroplasticity → Each daily micro-shift, from an affirmation to a successful craving resistance, sculpts your brain toward calm, confident sobriety.

Quick Win: Reframe a Negative Thought Today

1. **Catch a negative thought:** For example, *I'll never handle social events without drinking.*

2. **Challenge it:** Is it absolutely true? Have you ever managed a social event sober?

3. Replace it: *I'm learning new ways to socialize confidently. Each sober event strengthens me.*

Write down this reframe. You're literally documenting the moment you hacked your old mental loop and installed a more empowering script.

Your #Momhak365 Challenge: Start to Reprogram Your Mind in 7 Days

For the next week, commit to:

Three Affirmations Daily

Include your Personal Power Affirmation ("I am strong and relaxed thriving in sobriety") and your custom Pain–Pleasure Affirmation.

Pain–Pleasure Check

- Each morning, glance at your short list of painful consequences from addiction vs. the joys of sobriety.

- Let that perspective guide your decisions throughout the day.

Track Mindset Shifts

- Note each time you catch yourself in negative thought loops.

- Write down your reframe. Observe how your self-talk evolves.

Over time, notice:

- **More Confidence** – You'll start believing your new self-statements.

- **Reduced Cravings** – As pain associations grow around old habits, while new habits become pleasurable.

- **Better Emotional Mastery** – Emotions no longer feel unstoppable; you can name them, tame them, and choose a healthier path forward.

Bonus: Share at least one daily affirmation or reframe on social media or with a friend using **#Momhak365**. Witness how communal encouragement cements your transformation.

Momhak Moment: Your Thoughts Are Not Facts

Close your eyes, inhale for 4, exhale for 6, and envision:

- A tranquil river: see each negative thought as a floating leaf drifting past you.

- You are the observer on the bank, choosing which leaves to pick up and which to let float away.

- Affirm: "My thoughts do not define me—I select the beliefs that empower me."

Realize that **every moment** offers a choice: either cling to disempowering patterns or gently replace them with life-giving truths.

Looking Ahead: Chapter 7 – Daily Habits for Thriving

In the next chapter, we'll move from internal rewiring to **external routines.** You'll discover:

- A powerful morning ritual for mental clarity
- The habit-stacking formula for effortless success
- Why nutrition, sleep, and daily movement are essential to long-term sobriety

Remember: **Your thoughts create your life**. Now let's ensure that your **daily habits** anchor these changes, making your progress unstoppable.

CHAPTER 7: DAILY HABITS FOR THRIVING

WHAT YOU'LL DISCOVER

- Why daily habits form the bedrock of lasting transformation
- How morning and evening routines can supercharge your success
- The crucial roles of nutrition, sleep, and movement in stabilizing mood and reducing cravings
- Strategies to build consistency without relying solely on motivation

KEY INSIGHTS

- Small daily actions compound into massive changes over time
- A structured morning routine primes your brain for the day's challenges
- Quality sleep and whole-food nutrition keep your emotional and physical energy on track
- Habit stacking bridges new behaviors with existing routines for effortless adoption

YOUR TRANSFORMATION TOOLS

- Morning Rituals: Breathwork, affirmations, and movement to start strong
- Evening Wind-Down: Screen-free time, gratitude journaling, and relaxation
- Habit Loops: Build habits that stick via cues, routines, and rewards

• Micro-Commitments: Tiny, winnable steps that shape your future self

"No man is free who is not master of himself."
—Epictetus

Why Habits Matter More Than Willpower

You can have the most profound insights into addiction, the most inspiring success stories, or the most cutting-edge neuroscience—but if you don't translate these insights into **consistent daily actions**, the changes you crave remain elusive. Willpower alone is unreliable. It fluctuates with stress, mood, and even blood sugar levels. By contrast, well-structured habits function like autopilot: once installed, they require minimal mental energy to sustain.

The Power of Tiny, Consistent Steps

Self-help luminary James Clear calls this the "1% better" concept in his groundbreaking *Atomic Habits*. Become a fraction better each day, and by year's end, the cumulative gains are enormous. Instead of thinking, *I need to revamp my entire lifestyle right now,* ask, *What mini-habit can I adopt **today**?* This could be:

• Repeating affirmations while looking in the mirror while brushing your teeth

• Give yourself a burst of cold water at the beginning or in the middle of every shower

• Writing a single sentence in your journal each night

These might appear trivial, but they rewire your identity from the inside out. Once you experience that small win—like feeling more alert after a brief cold shower or more peaceful after a minute of gratitude—you reinforce a cycle of positive feedback in your brain.

Morning Routines: Begin with Purpose

Morning routines aren't just buzzwords from personal development gurus—they're a science-backed way to set a positive tone for the entire day. By consciously stacking a few healthy habits right after you wake up, you'll leverage the power of habit loops to align your mind and body toward success from minute one. Neglect the morning, and you often spend the rest of the day "catching up"—a recipe for stress, impulsive decisions, and, for many, craving triggers. Harness the morning, and you proactively shape your mental landscape long before external chaos hits.

Why Mornings Matters

Prime Your Brain: Cortisol (the "wake-up" hormone) peaks naturally in the first hour of being awake. Pairing it with activities like cold showers or affirmations can accelerate mental clarity.

Consistency: If you knock out healthy habits early, you're less likely to let the day's chaos push them aside.

Momentum: A strong, intentional start creates a ripple effect— when your morning feels "on track," you're more motivated to maintain positive choices throughout the day.

Sample Morning Ritual

Breathwork (10 to 15 minutes)

Tummo/Wim Hof: Start while still lying in bed with Tummo/Wim Hof breathing to energize your mind and body (refer back to Chapter 4 for technique details). This provides a natural boost in mood and alertness to carry you through your morning.

Affirmations (5 minutes)

Recite your Personal Power Affirmation or any short, powerful statement that fits the day and your mood. This can be integrated with your Tummo breathing: "I am relaxed, confident, and content thriving in sobriety." Remember to feel your affirmations in your body—imagine the warmth of self-assurance spreading from your chest down to your fingertips

Cold Shower or Cold Shot (30 seconds to 2 minutes)
Include a cold-water session in your regular shower to jolt your system awake and get a natural dopamine boost. Alternatively, move your shower to later in the day for an afternoon boost (flip back to Chapter 4 for details).

Micro-Journaling (5 to 15 minutes)
A quick note on your phone or in your journal. Keep it simple: "One thing I'm grateful for" or "My top intention for today."

Habit Stacking Example:

"Right after I brush my teeth, I do a 5-minute breathwork session."

"While I'm brewing coffee or tea, I recite one positive affirmation out loud."

If you have extra time in the morning, consider incorporating:

Light Movement or Yoga: Even 5 minutes of sun salutations or gentle stretching can help wake up your muscles and enhance circulation.

Hydration Ritual: A tall glass of water (with a squeeze of lemon if you like) rehydrates you after sleep and helps kick-start digestion. Best before your morning coffee or tea.

Natural Light Exposure: Stepping outside to catch a few minutes of morning sunlight not only boosts mood but also helps set your circadian rhythm.

Science Corner: Morning Routines & Dopamine

Establishing a consistent morning routine can regulate dopamine release throughout the day, stabilizing mood and reducing sudden cravings. The body thrives on predictable cues; when you start your day with deliberate self-care, you reinforce neural pathways that favor calm focus over impulsivity.

The Crucial Evening Wind-Down

Your nighttime routine is equally important. After a long day, it's easy to slip into mindless scrolling, late-night snacking, or anxious tossing and turning. But with just a little planning, you can create a soothing environment that sets you up for deep, restorative sleep—crucial for balanced hormones, emotional regulation, and preventing relapse and cravings.

Step 1: The Tech-Free Time

Stanford neuroscientist Andrew Huberman a emphasizes avoiding bright light (especially blue light from screens) in the 30 to 60 minutes before bed. This helps your body produce melatonin, the hormone that signals sleep.

- **Avoid** scrolling or streaming in bed—mindless screen time near bedtime can overstimulate your brain.

- **Preparing your clothes and work items** for the next day can also help you feel more organized and relaxed.

- **Alternative activities**: Instead of screen time, try winding down with a physical book, an audiobook, or a short breathwork session.

Why This Matters

When you bombard your eyes with screen light at night, you trick your brain into thinking it's daylight. This disrupts your circadian rhythm, the internal 24-hour clock guiding sleep-wake cycles. Compromised sleep often leads to poor impulse control the next day, weakening your defenses against cravings.

Step 2: Gratitude & Reflection

Gratitude Journaling: Write down a single thing that went well or a moment you appreciated during the day. This simple act shifts your mind into a calm, positive state, reducing sleep-disrupting anxiety.

Step 3: Soothing Movement or Yoga

Gentle Yin Yoga: Poses like **Child's Pose** or **Legs-Up-The-Wall** help reduce cortisol and invite a parasympathetic ("rest-and-digest") state. Even 5 minutes of slow stretching can lower physical tension built up over the day, easing you into deeper rest.

My personal evening wind-down begins with a shower that starts with an invigorating 2-minute cold burst, followed by a long, hot, relaxing rinse. Afterward, I practice a short yin yoga session—gentle, relaxed stretching that calms both my mind and body, helping me fall asleep faster and enjoy deeper rest.

If I'm still restless, I listen to an audiobook in bed that I've previously enjoyed, setting a 15 or 30-minute timer. If this disturbs your partner, you can buy inexpensive, Bluetooth, headband-style earbuds designed for sleeping. This shifts my mind from busy mode to storytelling time, easing me into sleep.

Body Scan in Bed

To close out your wind-down routine, try this simple yet powerful technique that helps transition both mind and body into deep rest:

Lie down, close your eyes, and mentally "scan" from your feet up to your head. Notice tension, then consciously relax each area.

This method, commonly taught in mindfulness-based stress reduction programs, can enhance sleep quality by calming the sympathetic nervous system (Kabat-Zinn, 2013).

Momhak Moment

Each night is an opportunity to reset. Choose to end your day with calm and intention and watch how tomorrow's dawn feels lighter.

Science Corner: Andrew Huberman's Sleep Strategies

Dr. Andrew Huberman of the *Huberman Lab Podcast* offers several actionable tips to optimize sleep:

Consistent Bed & Wake Times: A regular schedule synchronizes your circadian rhythm, making it easier to fall asleep and wake up energized.

Morning Light Exposure: Getting bright light in your eyes (ideally sunlight) within an hour of waking helps set your internal clock, improving nighttime melatonin release.

Avoid Bright Light at Night: Dim overhead lights and reduce screen brightness after sunset to prevent melatonin suppression.

Cool, Dark Room: Aim for a bedroom temperature around 65 to 70°F (18 to 21°C)—a cooler environment fosters deeper sleep.

Caffeine Curfew: He advises limiting caffeine to before noon or 2 p.m. at the latest. Elevated caffeine levels can linger in your system for 8 or more hours.

No Intense Exercise Close to Bed: High-intensity workouts within 2 hours of bedtime can spike adrenaline, making it harder to drift off. Opt for gentler evening movement like light stretching or yoga.

Why This Matters: Poor sleep can spike your stress hormones (like cortisol) and make you more vulnerable to cravings— dangerous territory if you're aiming for lasting freedom from addiction.

> *"Success is nothing more than a few simple disciplines, practiced every day."*
> —Jim Rohn, author of *The Art of Exceptional Living*

Midday Resets: Maintaining Momentum

So far, we've covered mornings and evenings in detail, but what about those critical midday hours? Many people find their resolve dips in the late afternoon, especially after a stressful workday or a conflict at home. A few well-placed micro-habits can keep you on track:

Quick Midday Strategies

Midday Breathing Break (2 to 5 minutes)

Use Mindful Breathing to reset. Pause and take 10 slow breaths, perhaps using the 4–6 pattern (Chapter 4), lengthening the exhale to calm your nervous system.

Hydration Check

Keep a large water bottle at your desk or in your bag. A great idea is to add cucumber for flavor.

Why It Matters: Mild dehydration can mimic hunger or fatigue, sometimes triggering the urge for a quick fix like sugary snacks or caffeine. Staying hydrated helps you differentiate real cravings from simple thirst.

Micro-Movement

Stand and stretch, or walk a lap around your office or block, do 10 squats, or hold a 30-second plank.

These micro-movements reduce stress and boost mood. Over a week, these small breaks add up, helping you maintain a level emotional keel.

Mind Hack

If an anxious thought appears—like *I need a drink to handle this stress*—spot-check it. Ask, *Is this real, or is it just a habit?* Then replace it: *I can handle stress. I choose a better response.*

Healthy Snack Prep

If you're prone to afternoon hunger, have snacks like carrot sticks, fruit, or a handful of nuts ready. By choosing nutrient-dense whole foods instead of junk, you reinforce the habit of fueling your body in ways that support your sobriety and mental clarity.

Incorporating these midday resets ensures that your morning momentum doesn't fizzle when life's stresses peak.

Whole-Food Nutrition for Daily Balance

Why Whole Foods Over Processed Ones?

What you eat has a direct impact on how you feel—physically, emotionally, and mentally. In my own recovery, shifting to a mostly whole-food, plant-based diet made a massive difference. I'm not rigid about it, and you don't have to be either. The key is simplicity: whole, minimally processed foods that support healing—not the ultra-processed stuff that mimics the highs and lows of addiction. The goal isn't perfection. It's alignment—choosing food that stabilizes your blood sugar, balances your mood, and supports your dopamine system. Whether your plate is entirely plants or includes some animal products, what matters most is that your meals are made of real, recognizable ingredients.

Why Avoid Highly Processed Foods?

- **Blood Sugar Spikes:** Ultra-processed carbs can create rapid highs and lows, leading to mood swings and intense cravings.

- **Nutrient Gaps:** Processed items are often stripped of fiber, vitamins, and minerals that your body and brain need to stay balanced.

- **Addictive Additives:** Many packaged foods are engineered to hit your reward system hard—blending sugar, salt, and fat in a way that's eerily similar to addictive substances.

Rule of Thumb: If it has a long ingredient list full of unpronounceable names, it's likely not supporting your recovery. Choose whole grains, legumes, fresh or frozen vegetables, fruits, nuts, seeds, and—if you eat animal products—stick to whole forms like steak, fish fillets, chicken breast, or oysters over things like deli meat, sausages, or frozen nuggets.

Building a Whole-Food Plate

Vegetables & Fruits: Fill about half your plate with colorful, seasonal produce.

Whole Grains or Starchy Veggies: Think brown rice, quinoa, oats, potatoes, sweet potatoes, or squash.

Protein Source: Beans, lentils, tofu, tempeh—or a clean, whole cut of meat or fish if that works for you.

Healthy Fats: Add avocado, nuts, seeds, or a drizzle of extra virgin olive oil or flaxseed oil for balance and satisfaction.

Quick Meal Prep Tips

Batch Cooking: Cook a large pot of quinoa or lentils once a week to simplify mealtimes.

Frozen Fruit & Veggies: They're often just as nutritious as fresh, and they save time without sacrificing quality.

Flavor Without the Junk: Experiment with herbs, spices, garlic, ginger, lemon, and vinegar to create delicious meals without resorting to processed sauces or sweeteners.

Mood & Energy Benefits

Whole foods help regulate your blood sugar, which keeps your energy steady and your mood more stable. When your body isn't swinging between highs and crashes, you're far less likely to reach for a sugary snack, a drink, or anything else to soothe discomfort.

Science Corner: Food, Dopamine & Craving Control

Dr. Andrew Huberman highlights that a steady, nutrient-dense diet helps regulate dopamine levels—crucial for maintaining focus, motivation, and impulse control during recovery. When dopamine is stable, cravings are easier to manage, and long-term brain health is better supported.

This isn't just about food as fuel—it's about food as chemistry. A diet rich in whole foods—fruits, vegetables, whole grains, and healthy fats—provides the nutrients your brain needs to regulate mood, balance blood sugar, and reduce the drive to self-soothe with substances.

In contrast, diets high in refined sugar and processed foods are linked to mood instability and emotional turbulence—exactly the conditions that make relapse more likely.

By eating with intention, you're not just nourishing your body—you're also reinforcing your recovery at the neural level.

Momhak Moment

Your daily plate is your daily vote—for higher energy, sharper focus, and fewer cravings.

Habit Stacking & Micro-Commitments

We've covered **habit stacking**—linking new behaviors to existing routines—to make them automatic (Clear, 2018). But what if you still feel overwhelmed? Try **micro-commitments**: so small they're almost laughable, but still incredibly helpful.

Examples of Micro-Commitments

A Single Stretch: Right after you stand up from your desk, do one forward fold or overhead reach.

One-Minute Journaling: Even a single sentence about your emotional state counts.

15-Second Cold Blast: Instead of a full-minute cold shower, start with 15 seconds.

30 Seconds of Deep Breathing: If you can't muster a 5-minute session, do 30 seconds.

These micro-commitments often evolve organically into longer sessions once you're in motion. And remember: The hardest part is initiating, not sustaining.

Quick Win: Set Your Stack for Tomorrow

Pick one daily habit you already do—like brushing your teeth or pouring your morning coffee–and decide what tiny action you'll stack onto it tomorrow. Write it down, or set a quick phone reminder. It could be one 4–6 breath, a single affirmation, or a 10-second stretch. That's how new neural pathways start—with one intentional link.

Building Consistency Without Motivation

Motivation is fickle. Some days, you wake up raring to go; others, you can't drag yourself out of bed. Systems outperform motivation because they run on cues and routines, not fleeting emotional highs.

The Habit Loop (Cue → Routine → Reward → Rewire)

Cue: A situational trigger (e.g., hearing your alarm, finishing lunch, or brushing your teeth)

Routine: The action you want to adopt (breathing, journaling, micro-mindfulness)

Reward: A small but immediate sense of accomplishment or relief—like checking off a task, feeling your mood lighten, or simply telling yourself "Great job!"

Rewire: Over repeated cycles, your brain cements this behavior as the default

Example:

Cue: Brushing your teeth in the morning

Routine: Inhale for 4 seconds, exhale for 6 seconds. Repeat 3 times

Reward: A quick mental pat on the back ("I'm starting the day centered!")

Rewire: After 3 or 4 weeks, you'll do it on autopilot

The Role of Social Accountability

Human beings thrive on social connection. Even mild accountability—like telling a friend or online group you'll do 2 minutes of yoga daily—can double your follow-through odds. If you've ever joined a workout buddy or a study group, you know the effect: You show up because someone else is waiting for you.

Ways to Tap Accountability
Partner Up
Recruit a friend, spouse, or coworker to commit to a shared habit. Maybe you both pledge to walk for 15 minutes or endure a cold shower daily.

Join a Community
Whether a local yoga studio, an online forum, or a simple text group, communal encouragement fosters resilience.

Public Declarations
Publicly stating intentions (like a social media post or group chat) significantly increases completion rates.

Momhak Moment
When others expect you to show up, you discover strength you didn't know you had.

Putting It All Together: A Day in the Life

Morning (30 to 45 minutes total)
Breathwork & Affirmations (10 mins)
Tummo breathing with affirmations and mindfulness during breath holds. "I am clear-headed and strong, thriving in sobriety."

Cold Shower (1 or 2 mins)
Begin with a 30-second cold burst, or start lukewarm and gradually drop the temperature.

Micro-Journal (5 mins)

Note your top intention for the day: "Today, I prioritize calm and kindness."

Midday (2 to 5 minutes each break)

- 1 minute of breath control every time you feel stress spiking

- Quick walk around the building or block

- Healthy snack/hydration check

Evening (15 to 30 minutes)

Tech-Free Wind-Down Time (At least 30 mins before bed)

Dim the lights, put away devices

Gratitude Journal (5 mins)

Note one win of the day, no matter how small

Gentle Movement or Body Scan (5 to 10 mins)

Yin yoga, mild stretching, or scanning from your toes to your head

Nighttime Sleep (7 to 9 hours)

- Keep your bedroom cool and dark

- Maintain a regular bedtime

- Avoid caffeine after 2 p.m.

Sustainability: Start small. If 45 minutes each morning sounds impossible, do 5 to 10 minutes. Let success breed success.

Chapter 7 Summary: Daily Habits for Thriving

Core Message

Your daily habits are the foundation of your transformation. Small, consistent routines—especially in the morning and evening—create momentum and make lasting change effortless.

Key Lessons

Small, Intentional Habits Lead to Massive Long-Term Change

Consistency trumps intensity. Don't aim for a radical overhaul overnight.

Structured Routines Anchor Your Day

A purposeful morning sets a positive tone; a mindful evening ensures deep rest.

Whole-Food Nutrition and Quality Sleep

Steady energy, balanced mood, and fewer cravings are direct payoffs of a nutrient-dense diet and solid rest.

Habit Stacking & Accountability

Integrate new behaviors into familiar cues, and let social support supercharge your commitment.

Your #Momhak365 Challenge: Build One New Habit This Week

For the next 7 days, commit to a new habit in one of these areas:

Morning Ritual: Breathwork, stretching, journaling, or hydration.

Evening Wind-Down: Screen-free time, gratitude journaling, stretching, or deep breathing.

Nutrition Focus: Swap one processed food for a whole, nutrient-dense option.

Sleep Optimization: Set a bedtime and stick to it for the full week. If you miss a day, resume immediately—no need for a guilt spiral.

Bonus: Share your new habit in the **#Momhak365** community. Seeing others' journeys can inspire fresh ideas or remind you that you're not alone when challenges arise.

Mindful Moment: See Who You're Becoming

- Close your eyes. Take a deep breath in for 4 seconds, then exhale for 6.

- Imagine yourself 6 months from now, thriving in a life built on strong, daily habits.

- See yourself waking up refreshed, eating nourishing food, handling stress with ease.

- Every small habit you build today is shaping this future version of you.

Looking Ahead: Social Challenges & Setting Boundaries

Chapter 8 tackles one of the biggest hurdles to sobriety: navigating social pressures, dealing with peer influence, and setting clear boundaries without alienating friends or family. You'll discover:

- How to say "no" gracefully

- The "no" script for awkward situations

- Ways to build a support system that strengthens your transformation

Habits shape your future—and your social environment can either reinforce them or tear them down. Let's make sure that your relationships and social circles align with your thriving new life.

CHAPTER 8: MASTERING SOCIAL CHALLENGES, OVERCOMING RELAPSE RISKS & BUILDING YOUR SUPPORT SYSTEM

WHAT YOU'LL DISCOVER

- How to handle social situations without feeling pressured to drink or use other substances
- The power of boundaries, scripts, and exit strategies for navigating triggers
- Why relapses happen—and how to recover quickly without guilt
- An expanded look at the role of THC in recovery: tool or trap?
- How to build a strong support system that reinforces your transformation

KEY INSIGHTS

- Social triggers are inevitable—the right preparation makes all the difference
- Confidence comes from having a plan before you enter high-risk environments
- Relapse isn't failure—it's data that refines your strategy
- THC can be bridging or binding—its impact in recovery is deeply individual
- Your tribe matters—the people around you can either accelerate or undermine your progress

TRANSFORMATION TOOLS

- "No" Script Exercise: Craft a simple, confident refusal for offers of alcohol or substances

- Emergency Reset Plan: A quick, step-by-step guide to bounce back after slip-ups

- Community Building: Methods to find or create the supportive relationships you need

- THC Decision Matrix: A framework for deciding whether cannabis is helping or hindering your recovery

"The key is to keep company only with people who uplift you, whose presence calls forth your best."
—Epictetus

Navigating the Noise

The journey to lasting freedom isn't just about you—it's also about the environments, people, and habits surrounding you. Whether you're navigating social events loaded with triggers, grappling with a slip-up, questioning the role of THC, or seeking a tribe of supporters, this chapter aims to equip you with tools for every scenario. As you'll see, proactive preparation is the difference between feeling overwhelmed and feeling in control.

Over time, your preferences for where—and with whom—you spend your time will likely shift. What once felt fun or normal, like hanging out in a pub every night, may start to feel draining, awkward, or simply out of alignment with your new priorities. That's not a loss—it's growth. As you evolve, your environment will, too. This chapter helps you navigate that transition without guilt or isolation.

Why Social Triggers Are Hard (& How to Handle Them)

Picture this: You're at a party, music is blasting, and everyone's passing around drinks. A few friends nudge you, urging you to have "just one." Or maybe it's happy hour after work, and you sense your old cravings flaring up. These aren't just hypothetical situations—they're real-world tests that can make or break your progress.

Typical High-Risk Scenarios

Parties & Bars: Peer pressure can be intense, especially if your social group traditionally bonds over alcohol.

Celebratory Events (Weddings, Holidays): Alcohol is often deeply woven into the festivities.

Stressful Gatherings: Family reunions or corporate events can unleash emotional triggers, from unresolved tension with relatives to workplace anxiety.

Preparation is your first defense. Walk into these events with a game plan: have an exit strategy if things get too intense, hold a non-alcoholic drink so that people don't constantly offer you one, or bring a supportive friend who "has your back."

"When I got sober, I thought giving up [alcohol] was saying goodbye to all the fun and all the sparkle, and it turned out to be just the opposite. That's when the sparkle started for me."
—Mary Karr

Why a Game Plan Matters

When you anticipate these scenarios, you can walk in with clarity. It's essential to:

Pre-set Boundaries: For instance, decide on a 60-minute time limit or commit to a non-alcoholic beverage.

Visualize Success: Picture yourself confidently turning down a drink or stepping outside for a breath break if tension spikes.

Enlist Support: Maybe you bring a trusted friend who understands your sobriety goals.

Momhak Moment

You don't have to avoid parties—you just need to show up with your own blueprint for success.

Boundary-Setting: The "No" Script & Exit Strategies

Boundaries protect your progress. Imagine them like invisible guardrails on a winding road—they don't limit your journey; they prevent you from tumbling off the cliff.

The "No" Script Exercise

1. Pick a Realistic Social Setting

Let's say you're going to a friend's house party next weekend.

2. Write Down a Refusal

This must be simple enough to remember under stress.

Examples:

"I'm good with what I have, but thanks for offering!"

"I'm taking a break from alcohol right now—just focusing on my health."

"I appreciate it, but I'm trying out these mocktails. They're good—have you tried them?"

3. Practice Aloud

Repetition cements neural pathways, making your script automatic when pressure arises.

4. Visualize Execution

Close your eyes, imagine the scenario, and say your script in your mind.

Goal: To feel natural saying "no" so that you won't freeze up in real-time.

Quick Win: Your Boundary Words

When you think about successfully holding a boundary in a social situation (like saying "no" confidently), what positive feelings come to mind? Quickly jot down 3- to 5 words (e.g., calm, confident, clear, grounded, respectful, proud, etc.). Circle the one that resonates most strongly with you today.

Exit Strategies

Time Limit: "I'll stay for one hour, then head out."

Driving: Park so that you aren't blocked in—the ease of leaving reduces social friction.

Buddy System: If you have a friend also avoiding alcohol, agree on a code phrase for leaving together.

It's okay to leave without a big goodbye: If the energy shifts or things start getting out of hand, quietly stepping out is often the best move. Most people won't even notice, and those who do will likely understand. A quick text to a friend still at the event lets them know that you're safe, and it avoids any unnecessary concern.

Case Study: Paul's 45-Minute Rule

A 32-year-old marketing manager discovered that corporate happy hours triggered intense cravings. He set a strict 45-minute window for these events—just enough time to mingle, then politely head home. Over months, his coworkers grew accustomed to his early departures. He found that limiting his exposure allowed him to feel in control and less anxious about potential slip-ups.

Explore the Evolving World of Alcohol-Free Beverages

One of the best ways to blend in socially (while staying sober) is to experiment with non-alcoholic drinks that taste great.

DIY Sodas & Mocktails: A SodaStream (or similar device) lets you craft carbonated water with fruit, herbs, and natural flavors.

Craft Mocktails: Bars and restaurants increasingly offer non-alcoholic versions of classic drinks—like virgin mojitos, virgin Bloody Marys, and more. Don't be shy about asking for something creative and booze-free.

Alcohol-Free Beer, Wine & Spirits: The market for alcohol-free beer, wine, and even "whiskey alternatives" has exploded, offering sophisticated flavors minus the buzz.

Why It Helps: Holding a glass that looks like everyone else's beverage can reduce social awkwardness. Plus, you won't feel deprived if you're sipping on something tasty and refined.

When I first started going to parties and bars sober, I discovered a small but powerful trick: **Always keep a drink in hand**—in my case, a cranberry soda. It's delicious, it looks like a cocktail, and at some bars, you even get free refills. This simple move helped me blend in without the awkwardness of constantly saying, "I'm not drinking."

At a friend's birthday BBQ, I gripped my cranberry soda as though it were a shield. Sure enough, people assumed it was a mixed drink, and the usual C'mon, have a beer!" comments barely came my way. But when someone *did* press me, I gave a small lift of my glass and said my pre-rehearsed line: "Thanks, I'm good with what I've got." That subtle gesture—with just a casual raise of the drink—was enough to signal I was already taken care of, and the moment passed without awkwardness. That moment showed me half of the fear was in my head: once I had a plan—and a tasty soda—I could stand my ground without drawing unwanted attention or feeling deprived. It was a small but empowering win that kept me confident and craving-free the entire night.

Remember, though, to use these alcohol-free drinks with caution! While they may seem like a harmless alternative, their resemblance in taste, smell, and ritual to actual alcohol can trigger cravings or even psychological relapse for some. For many in early recovery, these beverages blur the line between sobriety and old habits—so be honest with yourself about whether they support your healing or quietly keep you tethered to the past.

When Relapse Strikes: Recovery Without Shame

A slip-up isn't the end of your journey. Contrary to what some may believe, relapse is often a data point, not a moral failing. Yes, it can be heartbreaking, frustrating, or embarrassing—but it can also clarify what triggers still need your attention. I quit drinking more times than I can count! Some mornings, I'd pour out whatever beer I had left, determined to stop for good—only to find myself at the liquor store by afternoon, convincing myself that I had justification to drink for just one more day.

I remember convincing myself at a friend's wedding that I could handle just "one glass of champagne" after months of sobriety. Within a week, I was back to my daily 15-pack. That was the moment I realized that for me, "just one" was never just one—it was the beginning of a spiral. Learning how my brain processed those triggers was the lightbulb moment that changed my entire recovery path. Instead of seeing it as a failure, I saw it as data—proof that I needed a game plan for situations like that. Now I always walk into social events prepared: I hold a non-alcoholic drink in my hand, practice my "no" script ahead of time, and have an exit strategy if the pressure becomes too much.

Relapse as Data, Not Failure

Relapse can feel like a crushing blow, but it's not the end of your story—it's information. A slip doesn't mean that you're broken or incapable of change. It means that there's something you still need to learn about yourself, your patterns, or your environment. When approached with curiosity instead of shame, relapse becomes a powerful teacher. Here's how to extract the lesson and get back on track stronger than before:

Reflect, Don't Ruminate

The first instinct after a relapse is often to spiral into guilt or self-blame. But instead of asking, *What's wrong with me?* try asking, *What exactly happened?* Get specific. What were you feeling—overwhelmed, lonely, stressed, restless? Who were you with? What time of day was it? What were you doing just before the moment you slipped? This isn't about assigning blame—it's about identifying patterns. Every data point helps you prepare better for next time.

Reverse-Engineer a New Plan

Once you've identified the conditions that contributed to the relapse, work backwards and build a better strategy. If poor sleep and high stress set the stage, focus on creating evening routines that promote rest and practices that reduce daily tension—like breathwork, movement, or saying no to overcommitments. If social pressure played a role, revisit your "no" script, rethink your boundaries, or plan your exits in advance. A relapse often exposes the weak points in your plan, so use that insight to reinforce them.

Re-Engage Accountability

One of the fastest ways to regain stability is to reach out. Text a sober friend, call your sponsor, or check in with a therapist or recovery group. The longer you wait, the more the shame narrative can take over. But when you share openly, you break that spiral. You remind yourself that you're not alone, and you activate your support network. Often, the moment you speak the truth is the moment your healing resumes.

Momhak Moment

Every mistake holds a message. Treat a setback like a teacher, and your relapse becomes the foundation for your strongest comeback yet.

Emergency Reset Plan

Recovery Checklist

1. **Immediate Contact**: Reach out to a supportive friend, sponsor, or counselor.
2. **Revisit Affirmations**: Remind yourself of the Pain-Pleasure Principle (refer back to Chapter 6). Massive pain from the old habit, massive pleasure in sobriety.
3. **Schedule a Counseling Session**: If professional help has been part of your plan, now's the time to re-engage.
4. **Reflect & Adjust**: Journal the circumstances around the relapse—time of day, emotional state, social setting, etc. Adjust your strategy for the next time.

Bounce-Back Strategies

Visualize the Next Challenge: Take 5 minutes daily to imagine a high-risk scenario and how you'll respond differently. This mental rehearsal builds "muscle memory" for sober decision-making.

Seek Peer Feedback: In group therapy or online recovery forums, share your relapse story. Ask others, "How did you handle a similar situation?" Collective wisdom can reveal coping methods that you haven't tried yet.

Double Down on Self-Care: Relapses often coincide with lapses in self-care—like poor sleep, neglected exercise, or pent-up stress. Make a checklist of your daily self-care essentials (e.g., 10 minutes of Tummo breathing with affirmations, a healthy breakfast, or an evening wind-down routine). Sometimes, revamping daily habits can fortify you against the next wave of cravings.

THC in Recovery: Bridging or Binding?

THC presents a nuanced debate in addiction recovery. Some see it as a lesser evil that helps them detach from harder substances, while others find that it morphs into another chain holding them back (Lembke, 2021).

I'll share my experience with it, but let me be clear: THC is *not* a cure-all, nor is it for everyone. If you find yourself using it to avoid emotions rather than process them, it might be a sign that it's not serving you.

The Science of THC & The Brain

Cannabis interacts with the endocannabinoid system, especially CB1 receptors linked to mood, appetite, and dopamine regulation. Moderate amounts of THC can induce relaxation, mild euphoria, or pain relief. But heavy or prolonged use can:

- **Reduce motivation** (sometimes called "amotivational syndrome")

- **Trigger anxiety or paranoia** in predisposed individuals

- **Lead to psychological or physical dependence**, especially in those genetically susceptible (NIDA, 2021)

Potential Transitional Aid

- **Stress Relief**: Some find that THC soothes anxiety or aids sleep in early sobriety from harsher substances

- **Appetite & Nausea Control**: Those dealing with withdrawal or medication side effects might benefit in the short term

- **Social Pressure Buffer**: Holding a joint or vape can reduce peer pressure to drink, albeit substituting one substance for another

Emerging Risks

- **Dependency**: Cannabis use disorder (CUD) is recognized by mental health professionals, affecting around 30% of cannabis users at some point (NIDA, 2021).

- **Polydrug Use**: People who continue using THC might be more tempted to return to alcohol or combine substances.

- **Emotional Avoidance**: If THC is used to numb rather than heal underlying issues, the root triggers remain unaddressed.

THC Decision Matrix

Question	High-Risk Answer	Potentially Safe Answer
Why am I using THC?	To escape or avoid my emotions.	To manage a legitimate medical condition.
How often do I use it?	Daily or multiple times a day.	Occasionally, with specific purpose.
How does it affect my progress?	Increases anxiety or apathy.	Reduces my cravings or helps me function.
Do I crave it when it's unavailable?	Yes, I get anxious or irritable.	No, I can easily take it or leave it.
Have I consulted a professional?	No, I'm winging it on my own.	Yes, I've spoken to a therapist/doctor.

If multiple answers are in the high-risk column, you may be substituting one dependency for another.

If your usage is on the safer side—sporadic, mindful, and guided by medical or therapeutic input—it might be a short-term tool.

I went back and forth between daily THC use and complete abstinence, trying to find the balance. At first, it seemed like a harmless substitute—something to take the edge off without the destructive consequences of alcohol. But over time, I noticed a pattern: my motivation dipped, my clarity dulled, my overall stress levels increased and the drive to push myself faded. It wasn't an immediate crash like alcohol but rather a slow, creeping inertia. Eventually, I had to be brutally honest with myself—was THC truly helping me move forward, or was it just another anchor keeping me in place?

That's not to say that this will be everyone's experience. Biology, mental health, and personal circumstances all play a role in how cannabis affects recovery. For some, it may serve as a helpful tool; for others, it can become another cycle of dependence. The key is to evaluate it honestly—without rationalization or denial. If it's enhancing your life, that's fantastic. But if it's keeping you stagnant, it might be time to reassess.

Individualized Decision

No universal "yes" or "no" applies. Some find that THC is a gentle crutch to exit more destructive habits; others slip into daily, heavy use that stalls growth.

Honest Self-Assessment: Ask yourself, *Am I using THC to genuinely manage pain or stress, or am I running from uncomfortable emotions?*

Track Use & Impact: Notice if it impairs your focus, motivation, or leads to psychological dependence.

Consult Professionals: A therapist or recovery coach can provide an unbiased perspective.

Building a Resilient Support System

Your environment includes more than parties or bars—it's also the networks of friends, family, mentors, and communities that sustain you. A solid support system can drastically reduce relapse risk and supercharge your sense of belonging.

Accountability Partners & Sober Allies
Friends & Family
Pick someone you trust who respects your journey—maybe a sibling who checks in weekly or a friend who also wants to quit drinking.
Sober Buddies
Another friend in recovery who resonates with your journey and understands the challenges. They might also be able to share tips you haven't considered.
Peer Mentors
More experienced individuals who overcame addiction can guide you around pitfalls.
Sober Coaches
Recovery coaches (sometimes called sober coaches or sobriety mentors) provide structure, motivation, and personalized guidance, which is especially helpful if you're navigating early sobriety without formal programs.
Therapists or Counselors
Mental health professionals can help you unpack deeper issues behind addiction, manage anxiety or trauma, and build emotional resilience, giving you tools that go beyond just staying sober.

Safe Spaces & Online Communities
Reddit or Dedicated Forums
Subreddits like r/StopDrinking or r/leaves (for weed cessation) operate 24/7, so you can find quick support any time you're struggling.
SMART Recovery Meetings
Science-based group sessions focusing on self-empowerment and CBT.
12-Step Fellowships (AA, NA, CA)
Traditional but time-tested and largely successful. While the spiritual aspect may not appeal to everyone, many find fellowship and accountability helpful.

Sober Events & Classes
Yoga studios, running groups, or creative workshops often provide social connection without the pressure to drink.

Momhak.com
Consider the online Momhak community (#Momhak365, Momhak.com) as an accessible source of connection and shared experience.

The Power of Recovery Fellowships
Group-based recovery programs, like SMART Recovery or traditional 12-step communities, offer face-to-face and online meetings where you can discuss challenges in a confidential, supportive environment. While not everyone resonates with the same group culture, many find tremendous benefit in connecting with others who've battled similar addictions. Consistent fellowship attendance can significantly reduce relapse rates by fostering accountability, empathy, and shared coping strategies.

Momhak Moment
Alone, you can become discouraged. But linked to a supportive tribe, your resolve multiplies.

Service & Contribution
Volunteering or mentoring can be a hidden secret to long-term sobriety. Helping others:

- **Shifts Focus**: From your cravings or anxieties toward empathy and contribution

- **Boosts Self-Worth**: Realize that your experiences can uplift someone else's journey

- **Fosters Deeper Bonds**: You're joining communities of caring individuals, forging friendships that transcend surface-level small talk.

- **Deepens Your Own Growth:** Teaching or mentoring others reinforces the lessons you've learned, helping you internalize your tools and strategies on a deeper level. When you explain a concept—like reframing a craving or building a morning routine—you strengthen your own understanding and make it part of your identity.

Chapter 8 Summary: Mastering Social Challenges & Building Your Support System

Core Message

You don't have to hide from social situations or walk on eggshells. With clear boundaries, exit strategies, a considered stance on THC, and a supportive network, you can handle any environment without risking your progress.

Key Lessons

Social triggers are unavoidable—but a plan is your armor.

A relapse is data, not a moral failing. Study its causes, refine your strategies, and move forward.

THC can be either bridging or binding—you decide if it's a lesser evil or another cage.

A robust support system—whether friends, online allies, or mentors—magnifies your ability to stay sober.

Quick Win: Create Your "No" Script

Prepare for social situations by practicing a simple, confident way to refuse a drink.

Choose a response that feels natural to you:

- **Polite but firm:** "I'm good with what I have, thanks."

- **Direct:** "I don't drink anymore—it's the best decision I've ever made."

- **Lighthearted:** "I've had enough drinks for a lifetime!"

Practice saying it out loud and visualize yourself using it in a real-life situation.

Your #Momhak365 Challenge: Set One Social Boundary

For the next 7 days, commit to at least one of these boundary-setting actions:

- Decline a drink with confidence using your "no" script.

- Choose an alcohol-free drink to bring to social events.

- Set a time limit for a social event—leave when you feel in control.

- Let a supportive friend know about your decision to stay sober.

Bonus: Share your "no" script or boundary success with **#Momhak365**. Celebrate each time you maintain control in a social setting.

Mindful Moment: Reclaiming Your Social Life on Your Terms

1. Close your eyes. Breathe in for 4 seconds, then exhale for 6.

2. Picture yourself at a social event—there's music, laughter, and "social norms", and yet you feel calm, in control, free from anxiety.

3. Sense the confidence in your posture as you politely decline offers and enjoy genuine conversation without numbing.

4. This reality is yours to claim, supported by boundary skills, self-knowledge, and a circle that respects your growth.

Looking Ahead: Finding Purpose & Meaning Beyond Sobriety

In Chapter 9, we move beyond just avoiding alcohol and start building a life that excites you. We'll explore:

- How to create an identity beyond addiction

- The power of movement, creativity, and service in fulfilling your life

- How to write your personal "Why Statement" to keep you focused

CHAPTER 9: FINDING PURPOSE & MEANING

WHAT YOU'LL DISCOVER

- Why "just not drinking" isn't enough—you need a bigger vision for life

- How to shift from avoiding addiction to actively creating a fulfilling future

- The power of identity shifts—you're *far* more than your past behaviors

- How movement, creativity, and service help fill the void addiction left behind

- Why it's OK to be not OK—and how to handle emotional dips

- Methods to discover your unique purpose beyond just "staying sober"

- How to craft and refine a personal "Why" Statement that fuels motivation

KEY INSIGHTS

- Sobriety isn't just the absence of substances—it's the presence of purpose

- Your identity shapes your actions; upgrading your identity drives healthier behaviors

- Movement, creativity, and acts of service restore dopamine in sustainable ways

- Emotional fluctuations are normal in recovery—acceptance is key to resilience

- A strong "why" clarifies decisions, making relapse less tempting

YOUR TRANSFORMATION TOOLS

- Identity Shift Exercise: Rewrite limiting labels and adopt empowering ones

- It's OK to Be Not OK: Accepting emotional ebbs and flows

- Movement & Creativity: Building natural rewards into daily life

- Service & Connection: Alchemizing personal pain into shared purpose

- "Why" Statement Creation: A concise, energizing mission that guides action

- Deep-Dive Purpose Exercises: Techniques to discover meaning beyond mere sobriety

"Man is a goal seeking animal. His life only has meaning if he is reaching out and striving for his goals."
—Aristotle

Beyond Avoidance: Why Purpose Matters

In the earliest stages of recovery, it's all about stopping—stopping the drinks, stopping the self-destructive cycle, stopping the denial. That's both vital and difficult. But if we remain stuck in "stop mode," life can feel like a gray vacuum—free from the old chaos but still missing a driving force.

The Problem with "Just Not Drinking"

Many discover that once their cravings subside, they're left wondering, "What now?" Without a substance dictating your time, you suddenly have massive open spaces in your schedule—and mental space formerly occupied by compulsive thoughts. This can spark feelings of restlessness, boredom, or even confusion about what life is supposed to look like now.

Momhak Moment
Once the noise of addiction fades, the real question emerges: What will you do with your clarity?

Why Purpose Beats Willpower
Research in positive psychology (Ryan & Deci, 2000) shows that humans thrive not by mere restraint but by engaging pursuits that satisfy innate needs—like competence, connection, and autonomy. Purpose is the anchor that aligns daily actions with something bigger, making long-term sobriety feel like a joyful project rather than a dreary obligation.

Defining a New Identity
Our identities basically come down to the mental labels we give ourselves. When we say, "I'm lazy," "I'm a failure," or "I'm just an addict," we're effectively programming our subconscious to act in alignment with that script. And neuroscience proves it: repeated self-views can carve neural pathways that influence behavior (Dweck, 2006).

Moving from Old Labels to Empowered Ones
Old Label: "I'm an addict."

Empowered Replacement: "I'm a resilient individual, focused on building the life I want."

Label Liberation
1. **List Unhelpful Labels:** "I'm broken," "I'm hopeless," "I'm unworthy."
2. **Challenge Them:** Are these facts, or just stories?

3. Replace With Growth-Focused Statements: "I'm learning to handle challenges with strength. I'm enough, right now."

Quick Win: Rewrite Your Identity

Think of one limiting label you've carried—maybe something like "I'm a screw-up," "I always relapse," or "I'm not strong enough." Now rewrite it into an empowering identity rooted in growth and possibility. Start with this format:

Old Label: "I'm _____."
New Identity: "I'm someone who _____."

Examples:
Old Label: "I'm a failure."
New Identity: "I'm someone who learns from every challenge and keeps growing."
Old Label: "I'm just an addict."
New Identity: "I'm a resilient person building a life I love."

Write it down. Say it out loud. Post it somewhere visible. This is how you begin living as your future self—today.

Your Personal Power Affirmation as a Compass

Your Personal Power Affirmation isn't just about reinforcing confidence—it's also a compass guiding your actions toward your highest self. As you shift your identity from "someone trying to quit" to "someone building a life they love," let your affirmation evolve with you. Keep it visible—on your phone, your mirror, or written in your journal. The more you see it, the more your mind will adopt it as truth.

Momhak Moment

Your future self isn't determined by old labels—it's shaped by what you consistently do today.

Quick Story: From Alcoholic in Recovery to Marathoner

A man who'd struggled with heavy drinking rebranded himself as "a marathoner in training." Overnight, his daily routine changed: he began running each morning because "that's what marathoners do." Within months, he gained not only improved fitness but also improved self-esteem. This identity shift felt more motivating and less limiting—he wasn't "just not drinking"—he was **becoming an athlete**.

It's OK to Be Not OK

Contrary to popular belief, being sober doesn't mean that you'll always feel fantastic. Some days bring bursts of energy and gratitude; others bring loneliness, stress, or anxiety. **Recovery is a journey, not an emotional straight line.** As Eckhart Tolle wrote in *The Power of Now*, "Accept—then act. Whatever the present moment contains, accept it as if you had chosen it."

Normalizing Emotional Waves

After periods of substance use, the brain's reward system and stress responses can get out of balance. Dr. Lembke explains that learning to sit with discomfort instead of trying to escape it is key to resetting the brain and breaking free from compulsive habits (2021). Each time you let uncomfortable feelings pass without numbing them, you strengthen your ability to handle stress.

Practical Steps for Handling Difficult Days

1. **Identify What You're Feeling:** Pause and name the emotions you're experiencing—like "I'm sad," "I'm lonely," or "I'm restless." Acknowledging emotions helps reduce their intensity and gives you more control over your response.

2. **Slow Your Breathing:** Use the 4–6 Mindful Breathing technique (see Chapter 4) for at least 3 cycles to calm your nervous system.

3. Write It Down: Jot down 1 or 2 sentences about why you feel off. Seeing it on paper can help you process and release emotional tension.

4. Reach Out: Text a friend, call a helpline, or connect with a supportive community. Sharing how you feel can lighten the emotional load.

5. Practice Self-Compassion: Tell yourself, "It's OK to be not OK. Emotions come and go. This feeling won't last forever."

Expecting to feel emotionally steady all the time sets you up for frustration. Ups and downs are part of the process; accepting them as normal helps you grow more resilient, and over time, you'll find that the urge to escape uncomfortable feelings starts to fade.

Momhak Moment

Emotions are waves—your role isn't to drown in them but to ride them to shore.

Discovering Core Values and Crafting a "Why" Statement

Once you've recognized that sobriety alone isn't the end goal, it helps to define what is. Core values are the internal GPS points guiding decisions. They answer the question, **"What really matters to me?"** Living in alignment with your core values creates a sense of purpose and makes long-term sobriety feel more like a meaningful project rather than a daily struggle.

Many people value health, family, creativity, adventure, or spiritual growth, while others find meaning in social justice, community building, or lifelong learning. Defining your values helps you shape a life that feels rewarding and fulfilling.

Find Your Core Values

Follow these steps to uncover your fundamental beliefs:

1. **Reflect on Peak Moments:** Think of a time when you felt truly alive or deeply fulfilled. What value was being expressed in that moment (e.g., growth, connection, nature)?

2. **Notice Anger Triggers:** We tend to become most upset when a deep conviction is violated. If dishonesty upsets you, honesty may be one of your core values.

3. **Write Down 3 to 5 Keywords:** From the list below, pick the values that resonate most with you. These will become the foundation for your "Why" statement.

Momhak Moment

Your values are your compass. They help you stay true even when the path feels uncertain.

List of Core Values

Below is a list of core values to help you get started:

Relationships & Connection

- Family
- Friendship
- Trust
- Love
- Community
- Belonging
- Compassion
- Loyalty

Personal Growth & Fulfillment

- Authenticity
- Self-Improvement
- Learning
- Mastery
- Creativity
- Curiosity
- Resilience
- Freedom

Health & Well-being

- Physical health
- Mental health
- Vitality
- Balance
- Self-care
- Nutrition
- Fitness
- Rest

Spiritual & Emotional Anchors

- Inner peace
- Mindfulness
- Gratitude
- Spirituality
- Forgiveness

Contribution & Service

- Helping others
- Generosity
- Justice
- Altruism

Adventure & Experience

- Exploration
- Fun
- Excitement
- New experiences
- Travel

- Acceptance
- Faith
- Presence

- Environmental care

- Playfulness

Work & Achievement
- Purpose
- Career success
- Financial stability
- Professional growth
- Ambition

Integrity & Character
- Honesty
- Courage
- Accountability
- Fairness
- Kindness
- Humility
- Respect

Nature & Environment
- Sustainability
- Connection to nature
- Adventure in the outdoors
- Environmental stewardship

"If you want to be happy, set a goal that commands your thoughts, liberates your energy, and inspires your hopes."
—Andrew Carnegie

Creating Your "Why" Statement

Once you've chosen your core values, it's time to craft a personal "Why" Statement. A strong "Why" gives you direction and motivation, especially when cravings or self-doubt surface.

Here's the "Why" Statement formula:

"I live to [core value] by [action or behavior] so that I can [impact or outcome]."

Examples:

- "I live to experience life fully by embracing each moment with curiosity so that I can stay grounded in the now."

- "I live to strengthen my mind by choosing discipline over distraction so that I can reclaim my freedom."

- "I live to lead by example by walking the path of recovery so that I can show others that freedom is possible."

- "I live to cultivate resilience by staying active and facing challenges head-on so that I can live with strength and confidence."

- "I live to make a difference by sharing my story and tools so that I can help others heal and rise."

Action Steps:

1. Choose 3 to 5 core values from the list above.

2. Craft a single "Why" Statement based on those values.

3. Write it down and place it somewhere you'll see it daily (e.g., your mirror, phone screen, or journal).

Your "Why" in Color: What color(s) do you associate with your "Why" Statement or your most important core value? Quickly jot down the color(s) and one word about why they resonate (e.g., "Green - growth, nature," "Blue - calm, clarity"). It's a simple way to connect emotionally to your purpose.

Movement as a Recovery Cornerstone

Physical activity can be both a core value (health, vitality) and a natural dopamine booster without the crash. Research shows that regular exercise can improve mood, reduce cravings, and support long-term recovery from substance use. Exercise helps regulate the brain's reward system, fosters resilience, and provides a healthy outlet for stress, creating forward momentum in your recovery journey.

Quick Win: Movement Mission

1. List 3 ways you can incorporate movement this week (e.g., walking 15 minutes daily, trying a gentle yoga class, or dancing in your living room).

2. Pick one and schedule it. Notice how you feel afterward, both physically and mentally.

I moved to Tofino (in British Columbia, Canada), a surfing hub, to immerse myself in the ocean, paddleboarding, and swimming. You don't need to relocate, but you can reclaim old hobbies and passions or explore new ones—like cycling, rock climbing, or martial arts—that align with your sense of curiosity.

Momhak Moment

Purpose is the light on the path, and your "Why" keeps your footsteps steady when the journey feels dark.

Expanding Purpose Beyond Sobriety: Key Approaches

1. Movement & Creativity

When you pursue enjoyable physical or creative activities, you create "clean dopamine." Let's say that you join a community dance class, paint, or learn guitar. The brain experiences healthy reward loops—without the downward spiral that substances bring. This is especially powerful if your old identity revolved around using or partying.

Deep Dive: Flow States

Psychologist Mihaly Csikszentmihalyi introduced the concept of "flow" as a state of total immersion in a challenging but achievable activity—like painting, writing, surfing, or even problem-solving. In his book *Flow: The Psychology of Optimal Experience*, Csikszentmihalyi explains that flow happens when your skill level is well-matched to the challenge at hand—difficult enough to engage you but not so hard that it causes frustration. In this state, time seems to disappear, your sense of self fades, and you become fully absorbed in the present moment.

Flow is powerful because it creates intrinsic rewards. Unlike artificial highs from substances, which often lead to a crash, flow generates a deep sense of satisfaction and meaning. Csikszentmihalyi argues that flow is one of the most reliable sources of happiness because it aligns with our natural drive for growth and mastery. He found that people who regularly experience flow report higher levels of life satisfaction and emotional well-being.

In recovery, flow can be a game-changer. Engaging in creative or active pursuits—whether it's playing music, hiking, cooking, or gardening—can naturally boost dopamine levels and create a sustainable sense of fulfillment. Flow helps shift your brain's reward system away from short-term, artificial stimulation (like substances or social media) and toward lasting internal satisfaction. If you've ever lost track of time while doing something you love— getting lost in a creative project, feeling fully present during a run, or being immersed in conversation—you've experienced flow. Incorporating more flow-inducing activities into your daily life not only enhances well-being but also builds resilience against cravings and emotional lows.

Example: A woman who quit heavy drinking found that daily pottery sessions calmed her mind. The tactile nature of clay, the focus on shaping forms, and the small creative triumphs replaced her old "happy hour" with a more sustainable form of happiness.

2. Service & Contribution

Purpose grows exponentially when shared. If you've ever helped a friend move, volunteered at a shelter, or coached youth sports, you know how fulfilling it can be. Service offers dual benefits: the recipient gains your support, and you gain a sense of meaningful connection.

Ways to Serve

- **Mentoring**: Many in recovery eventually mentor newcomers, sharing experiences and providing a supportive ear.

- **Volunteering**: Animal shelters, community gardens, soup kitchens—pick something you care about.

- **Creative Altruism**: If you're an artist, you can donate pieces to charity events. If you're a musician, offer free lessons to at-risk youth.

Peer Support & Volunteer Work in Recovery

Engaging in volunteer work or peer support roles can significantly enhance recovery outcomes. Peer support provides a sense of connection and accountability, while helping others fosters purpose and emotional fulfillment. People who actively participate in recovery communities or volunteer work often report stronger emotional resilience and higher rates of sustained sobriety. Helping others transcends "willpower" alone—it reinforces personal growth by creating a sense of belonging and purpose. When you support others in their recovery journey, you strengthen your own, turning personal progress into collective benefit.

Momhak Moment

When you lift someone else, you lift yourself. Healing isn't just about what you overcome—it's about who you help along the way.

3. Forgiveness & Turning Pain into Purpose

Psychiatrist and Holocaust survivor Viktor Frankl believed that our response to suffering shapes our destiny (Frankl, 1959). He endured unimaginable pain and loss in Nazi concentration camps, where he was stripped of his freedom, his family, and his dignity. But he discovered that even in the face of profound suffering, human beings have the freedom to choose their response. Frankl found that those who survived with their spirit intact were often those who could find meaning in their suffering. For him, that meaning came from helping fellow prisoners, offering comfort and hope despite the horror surrounding them.

Frankl's experience taught him that suffering itself is not the key to growth—it's the meaning we assign to it and how we respond that determines whether it becomes a source of strength or a source of despair. His work later inspired countless others to transform their own suffering into purpose, helping others find hope and resilience through difficult times.

The same principle applies in recovery. The pain of addiction and its consequences can feel overwhelming—but it also holds the potential for growth. When you process and release your pain, you create space to turn that experience into empathy, wisdom, and the ability to help others.

The Forgiveness Process

Acknowledge the Hurt: This isn't about excusing harm done; it's about freeing yourself from resentment's grip. Holding onto bitterness only deepens the wound.

Self-Compassion: Many people in recovery carry guilt or shame for past mistakes. Recognizing that you're more than your worst moments creates the space for healing.

Growth Perspective: Ask yourself, *How can my past struggles equip me to guide, support, or empathize with others?* Pain loses its hold when it becomes a tool for helping others.

Science Corner

Research from the University of Wisconsin-Madison found that forgiveness therapy significantly improves mental health outcomes for individuals in addiction recovery. A study by Lin et al. (2004) showed that participants who completed forgiveness therapy experienced reduced anger, depression, and anxiety, along with increased self-esteem and lower vulnerability to drug use. Forgiveness helped participants process unresolved pain, breaking the cycle of emotional distress that often fuels addictive behaviors. These findings underscore that learning to forgive—both yourself and others—can be a powerful tool for emotional healing and long-term recovery.

4. Stillness & Inner Connection

While not everyone identifies as spiritual or religious, finding time for mindfulness, reflection, or prayer can deepen your sense of meaning. A short daily practice—like mindful meditation, reading inspirational texts, or sitting quietly in nature—often recalibrates the mind, reminding you that life is more expansive than day-to-day anxieties.

Practical Spiritual Reflections

Nature Walks: Contemplate the rhythm of the seasons, the interconnectedness of life.

Gratitude Lists: Jot down three things you're grateful for daily. This simple act can shift perspective from lack to abundance (Emmons & McCullough, 2003).

Breath-Focused Meditation: Gently anchor your attention to each inhale and exhale. When your mind wanders, simply return to the rhythm of your breath.

Momhak Moment

Sometimes, stepping into quiet spaces of reflection clarifies your purpose more than any amount of activity.

Daily Actions for Purpose-Fueled Living

All the ideas above—movement, creativity, service, forgiveness— come alive when translated into daily or weekly habits. Instead of a vague notion of "find purpose," you integrate tangible routines that steadily deepen your sense of meaning.

Example "Purpose Day"
Morning (10 minutes)

- Read your "Why" Statement.

- Engage in 1 minute of Mindful Breathing, holding compassion for any emotions you wake up with.

Midday (15 minutes)

- Take a short walk to clear your head or engage in a creative micro-project (e.g., sketch, knit, or doodle a mind-map of ideas).

- Ask yourself, *How does today's to-do list align with my core values?*

Afternoon or Evening (30 to 60 minutes)

- Engage in a service-related activity—like checking in on a friend in recovery, volunteering at a local shelter, or simply helping a neighbor in need.

- Alternatively, dive into a hobby that sparks flow, such as painting, yoga, or learning guitar.

Night (5 to 10 minutes)

- Reflect on moments when you've felt alive or connected.

- Jot down 1 to 3 things you're grateful for.

- Reaffirm: "It's OK to be not OK if tough feelings appear. I'm still living my purpose."

Over weeks and months, these small purposeful actions compound, reshaping not just your habits but also your identity.

Vision Checkpoint

Remember the 5-month/5-year vision exercise from the Introduction? Now that you've explored identity, emotional acceptance, and purpose, revisit those early sketches of your future self. How do they align with the new practices you're developing?

Compare Then & Now:

- Have you begun adding movement to your routine?

- Are you more likely to reach out when sad rather than isolate?

- Do you notice fewer cravings, or at least an easier time riding them out?

Refine Your Goals:

- If something in your vision feels out of sync, adjust it. Recovery is fluid, and so are dreams.

- If you're more ambitious now, expand your goals—maybe you see yourself starting a small business or traveling to places you once only dreamed of.

Daily Visibility:

- Post your refined vision or "Why" Statement on a sticky note, your phone background, or a dedicated corner of your home.

- Glance at it when negativity creeps in, and let it ground you in your bigger aim.

Momhak Moment

Your vision is a living document. Allow it to grow with you as you rediscover your capacity for joy, courage, and empathy.

Deepening Purpose: Additional Exercises

Ikigai (Japanese Concept of "Reason for Being")

Ikigai is often depicted as the overlap of four circles:

- What you love

- What you're good at

- What the world needs

- What can support you financially (or at least not harm your stability)

While you don't need to follow the model rigidly, exploring these categories can spark fresh insights:

- **What do I love doing?** Think of childhood passions or current curiosities.

- **What am I good at?** This could be professional skills or personal traits (e.g., empathy, organizing).

- **What does the world around me need?** A local cause? Mentorship? Creative expression that uplifts?

- **How do I ensure that I'm stable financially or practically?** This might mean adjusting a hobby into a side pursuit or a career pivot.

Practical Tip: Sketch out a 2 x 2 grid or overlapping circles. Brainstorm each corner. Even small intersections can reveal ways to live with more meaning.

Internal vs. External Purpose

Internal Purpose: Personal growth, emotional clarity, spiritual practices, healing old wounds.

External Purpose: Serving community, building a family, creating something lasting for others.

We often find the strongest motivation when these converge— when our internal growth fuels external contributions, and vice versa.

Example: A man experiences internal healing through journaling his struggles. Over time, these journals become a blog that helps thousands facing similar challenges.

Breaking Down "Not OK" Feelings with Purpose

Despite all the purposeful planning, you'll still wake up sometimes feeling adrift. But this is where you can combine acceptance ("It's OK to be not OK") with one purposeful act. Even a small step— like sending a "thinking of you" note to someone who's hurting— can realign you with your deeper mission. The best antidote to gloom is often outward service or a forward-looking creative action.

"Whatever the present moment contains, accept it like you had chosen it. Always work with it, not against it. Make it your friend and ally, not your

enemy. This will miraculously transform your whole life.”
—Eckhart Tolle

Chapter 9 Summary: Finding Purpose & Meaning

Core Message

Ending self-destructive behavior is only part of the journey. Sobriety sparks a new frontier: building a life that resonates with your deepest values and aspirations. Through identity upgrades, acceptance of emotional ebbs and flows, and intentional daily actions—like movement, service, creativity, and reflection—you discover a sense of purpose that makes relapse less tempting and each day more meaningful.

Key Lessons

Sobriety Is a Springboard: Without a vision, sobriety can feel like empty space. Purpose fills that space.

Identity Shapes Behavior: Shifting from "I'm an addict" to "I'm a resilient, purposeful person" reshapes your subconscious roadmap.

It's OK to Be Not OK: Emotional waves are normal; acceptance with the added benefit of coping skills fosters lasting resilience.

Exercise & Service: Simple daily acts—like walking, volunteering, or helping a friend—rebuild healthy dopamine pathways and deepen your sense of meaning.

Keep Refining Your "Why": Purpose evolves as you grow. Let your mission remain flexible and adaptable.

Quick Win: Expand Your Identity

1. List old labels: "addict," "failure," "weak," "hopeless."

2. Cross them out.

3. Replace with growth statements:

- "I'm strong, healing, and growing daily."

- "I'm allowed off days, but my purpose remains."

Your #Momhak365 Challenge
Write or Refine Your "Why" Statement

1. Identify 2 or 3 Core Values: health, service, creativity, freedom, etc.

2. Visualize: Picture who you want to be in one year, and also in 5 years.

3. Condense to One Line: Example—"I live to experience life fully by embracing each moment with curiosity so that I can stay grounded in the now."

4. Read Daily: Morning and evening, or whenever negativity creeps in.

Track how this reframes your decisions. Feel free to share your "Why" Statement using **#Momhak365**—public or community-based accountability often strengthens commitment.

Mindful Moment: Embracing Purpose Amid Imperfections

1. Close Your Eyes: Inhale for 4 seconds, exhale for 6.

2. Visualize: Picture a scenario in which you woke up feeling "not OK." Imagine yourself pausing, breathing, and choosing a purposeful act—maybe going for a walk or journaling about gratitude.

3. Notice: Take note of how a small purposeful step transforms your mood. Let that calm or resolve spread through your body.

4. Accept: The path isn't perfect; it's human. Emotions fluctuate, but your deeper mission remains.

Looking Ahead: Thriving Beyond Sobriety

In Chapter 10, you'll move even further beyond simple avoidance of substances into sustainable growth and joy:

- Replacing old cravings with genuine passions

- How social support, movement, and creativity build a relapse-proof lifestyle

- Designing a future that evolves with you, keeping each day inspired

You're not "just not drinking"—you're building a life so fulfilling that you no longer feel the urge to numb out.

CHAPTER 10: THRIVING BEYOND SOBRIETY

WHAT YOU'LL DISCOVER

- How to shift from recovery into momentum—building a life that pulls you forward

- Why long-term success requires more than sobriety—it demands direction

- The role of movement, mastery, and meaning in rewiring your reward system

- How to create a lifestyle that energizes you—physically, mentally, and emotionally

- Daily habits that make relapse feel irrelevant—not just avoidable

KEY INSIGHTS

- Sobriety isn't the destination—it's the launchpad

- The best way to stay free from addiction is to fall in love with what comes next

- Passion, purpose, and movement create sustainable dopamine and resilience

- A growth-oriented lifestyle doesn't just protect your progress— it multiplies it

- Thriving means designing your life—not just avoiding your past

YOUR TRANSFORMATION TOOLS

- Passion Snapshot: Rediscover what lights you up—and take the first step toward it

- Movement Integration Plan: Create an exercise routine that boosts dopamine, focus, and joy

- Purpose Alignment: Anchor your daily habits to your personal "Why" Statement

- Tribe Building: Surround yourself with people who reflect and reinforce your growth

- Lifestyle Design Blueprint: Practical systems to structure your days for energy, purpose, and upward momentum

"The happiness of your life depends upon the quality of your thoughts."
—Marcus Aurelius

Momentum Over Maintenance

You've crossed a threshold and broken the loop… but now what? This isn't the chapter in which we talk about staying sober—it's the one in which you learn to thrive.

Recovery gives you back something you may not have realized was missing: *momentum*. You're no longer waking up in survival mode, dragging yourself out of bed and wondering if you'll make it through the day without slipping. Now you get to wake up and ask something far more powerful: **What do I want to build with this freedom?**

This is your permission slip to live big. To stop defining your life by what you've quit and start defining it by what you're creating. Because the truth is that the best relapse prevention isn't white-knuckled avoidance—it's a life so rich and exciting that the old cravings don't stand a chance.

"Recovery is not about never having a bad day. It's about learning how to live well in the midst of them."
—Unknown

This Is Where the Real Adventure Begins

In *Dopamine Nation*, Dr. Anna Lembke reminds us that the same pathways that were hijacked by substances can be rewired through movement, mastery, and meaningful connection. This chapter shows you how to do exactly that—not through rigid discipline but by engaging with the world in a way that floods your brain with **clean dopamine** and lights your spirit on fire.

Think of this as your **level-up chapter**. Not maintenance. Not management. *Momentum*. We'll explore how to channel your energy into passions, relationships, and routines that feed your growth—and how to make that growth feel natural.

This is about stepping into your next identity—not as "someone in recovery" but as a creator, a builder, a mover, a teacher, an athlete, an artist, or a leader. Whatever calls to you.

The work you've done up to this point has prepared you for this moment. You've cleared the weeds. Now it's time to plant the garden.

Momhak Moment

Your identity is no longer "someone running away from addiction." You're a creator, an explorer, and a builder of new possibilities.

Embracing Abundance Instead of Fear

Fear may get you sober—but it won't keep you growing. When you shift your mindset from avoiding relapse to pursuing a better life, everything changes. The human brain is wired for forward momentum. If you're constantly bracing for failure, you stay stuck in survival mode. But when you start chasing goals that excite you—learning a skill, building strength, helping others—you create a future that pulls you forward.

- **Reframe**: Each morning, instead of "I must avoid messing up," try, "I'm excited to see how I'll grow today."

- **Daily Nudge**: Place a sticky note or phone reminder that says, "I'm building a life that energizes and excites me."

Reclaiming Time & Energy—Discovering New Passions

Addiction doesn't just harm your body; it monopolizes your **time**, **money**, and **mental space**. Think of the hours spent using, recovering, or worrying about your next fix. Now that you're clear-headed, you have a previously "lost" resource: **abundant time** and **mental capacity**.

The Power of Free Time

Imagine you start each weekend without a hangover. Suddenly, those two days aren't about damage control—they're opportunities for new experiences. Or consider the **unclaimed moments**, like those 30 minutes before work that you once spent feeling anxious or hungover. Now you can channel that time into something uplifting: journaling, a short workout, a walk in nature, or simply relaxing and planning your day with intention.

Daily Log Tip

- For one week, jot down any new blocks of free time that appear because you're no longer "using" or "recovering."

- Dream about how you might fill those slots—5 to 15 minutes at a time. Short bursts can add up to big transformations.

Thriving Soundtrack

What's one song that makes you feel alive, energized, and excited about the future you're building? Write down the title and artist.

Consider adding it to a playlist you listen to during movement or creative time this week.

Replacing Old Obsessions with Healthy Ones

Many of us who struggled with substances have strong, persistent focus (sometimes called an "addictive personality"). But that same intensity can become an asset when channeled into healthy pursuits. Consider:

1. **Outdoor Adventures:** Hiking, kayaking, paddleboarding, or rock climbing. Nature challenges the body and soothes the mind.

2. **Artistic Passions:** Painting, sculpture, writing, content creating or photography. Creativity provides a dopamine lift and fosters self-expression (Csikszentmihalyi, 1990).

3. **Socially Engaged Hobbies:** Theater groups, team sports, choirs, dance classes, or martial arts—whatever you choose, group activities offer camaraderie and accountability.

4. **Skill Mastery:** Coding, woodworking, gardening—anything that requires practice and yields tangible results.

Making it Stick

Schedule: Many fresh interests fail because they remain indefinite. Pick a specific time, like "Every Thursday at 6 p.m., I go to pottery."

Minimal Gear: Buy or borrow just enough to feel committed. If you're trying yoga, invest in a decent mat. If you're learning guitar, purchase a reliable (but not necessarily expensive) instrument.

Share: Invite a friend to try your hobby with you or talk about it in a supportive forum. Public commitments often reinforce follow-through (Clear, 2018).

Why Movement Matters for a Thriving Future

Earlier chapters have touched on movement as a tool for managing cravings and stabilizing mood. But it's more than a temporary solution—it can be a **cornerstone** of your new lifestyle. According to Dr. Lembke, exercise is one of the few activities that provides sustained dopamine without the crash-and-burn effect of substances.

From Recovery Tool to Life Enhancement

A landmark paper in *The Lancet Psychiatry* found that regular exercise correlates with better mental health and resilience over time (Chekroud et al., 2018). For those in recovery, consistent movement can:

- **Regulate stress more effectively**, helping you stay grounded in challenging moments
- **Improve sleep quality**, making it easier to fall asleep and wake up restored
- **Stabilize mood**, reducing the emotional swings that often fuel cravings
- **Strengthen social bonds**, especially when practiced in groups like yoga classes, hiking clubs, or community sports

Shifting Your Mindset

Instead of seeing exercise as an optional chore, think of it as "plugging in" to a natural energy source. One that:

1. **Builds Physical Strength:** This encourages confidence in your body's abilities
2. **Centers the Mind:** Many forms of exercise—running, walking, yoga, swimming—can induce "flow" states
3. **Creates Social Bridges:** Fitness classes or sports teams can help you meet like-minded individuals

Building the Movement Practice

Morning Energy

- Start with simple stretching or a brief walk outside

- Optionally add gentle breathwork or affirmations (e.g., "I'm energized and looking forward to the day")

Midday Refresh

- If you have a desk job, take quick walking breaks, or 2 or 3 minutes of bodyweight exercises (like squats or push-ups)

- The surge in blood flow resets your focus and lifts your mood

Evening Exploration

- Sign up for a dance or martial arts class

- Explore local nature trails for a sunset walk with friends

Skill Development

- Set short-term goals (e.g., run a 5K, master 5 yoga poses, or learn to do a handstand)

- Track progress in a journal; it's motivating to see micro-improvements each week

Momhak Moment

Movement is more than burning calories—it's a daily reminder that your body is a source of freedom, not a cage held captive by old habits.

Action Step: Reclaim Your Curiosity

- Choose one form of movement you find appealing or at least intriguing

- Schedule it 2 or 3 times next week. A simple phone reminder—like "Wednesday 7 p.m. - 20-minute yoga flow"—increases follow-through

- Observe changes in your mood, energy, and outlook

Living On Purpose: Turning Vision Into Daily Practice

At this stage in your journey, you're no longer just avoiding the old—you're actively building the new. And that new life? It's not built on motivation alone. It's built on purpose.

Not the kind of abstract, once-a-year-on-a-vision-board kind of purpose, but something more immediate. Purpose that gets into your bones, that organizes your days and colors your choices. When you start living in alignment with what truly matters to you, momentum becomes natural.

This isn't about having your "life mission" perfectly figured out. It's about waking up with a reason—however small—and letting that reason guide you.

Let Purpose Guide Your Energy

You already know what lights you up. You've sketched the map with your "Why" Statement and clarified your core values. Now it's time to turn those insights into structure so that you're not just inspired occasionally but anchored daily.

Think of it like this: Your purpose is the compass, and your habits are the route. And every action is a step toward the life you're meant to build.

Here's how to bring it into motion:

1. Bookend Your Day with Intention

- **In the morning**, take 30 seconds to reconnect to your deeper reason for being. No need to overthink it—just pause and remind yourself, "Today, I live from…" followed by a keyword or phrase from your "Why" (e.g., compassion, creativity, or courage). Say it out loud or write it in your journal.

- **In the evening**, reflect briefly, "In what ways did I act from that place today?" No judgment—just awareness. This builds neural reinforcement and keeps your actions aligned.

2. Move with Meaning

Let your physical practices double as mindful ones.

- When walking, silently repeat your "Why" Statement as a rhythmic mantra.

- When doing Mindful Breathing or Cold Exposure, visualize the life you're working toward.

- When journaling or stretching, reflect on what gives your day meaning.

This subtle layering of intention into existing routines transforms them from maintenance into mission.

3. Audit Your Environment

Your lifestyle is a feedback loop. If it's designed unconsciously, it'll pull you into unconscious habits. But if it reflects your values, it'll continually guide you back to purpose.

Scan your calendar: Does how you spend your time reflect what matters to you?

Scan your space: Are there visual cues—quotes, photos, reminders—that bring your deeper values to the surface?

Scan your circle: Do the people closest to you reflect the direction you're going—or the one you left behind?

4. Redesign the Mundane

Purpose isn't just found in big goals—it lives in the ordinary, too. Doing the dishes, walking the dog, answering emails—all of it can be purposeful if connected to something larger.
Try linking small tasks to your greater values:

- "I clean my home to support my clarity and calmness."

- "I reply to this message with kindness because presence matters."

- "I cook this meal because nourishment is part of my self-respect."

This is how you stop grinding through your days and start **living** them.

A Day with Purpose in Motion

Morning: Quick breathing session + your Personal Power Affirmation and "Why" Statement

Midday: Outdoor walk with a silent affirmation or reflection

Afternoon: Engage in one task (work, service, connection) that reinforces your core values

Evening: Gentle movement (yoga, dance, or stretch) + write one sentence: "Here's how I lived on purpose today…"

Momhak Moment

Purpose doesn't have to be dramatic to be powerful. It just needs to be **present.** Bring it into your morning breath, your afternoon walks, and your bedtime thoughts. Let it weave through the quiet parts of your day—and watch how your life begins to rise to meet it.

Building Your Tribe & Sustaining Growth

Sobriety is powerful, but **community** supercharges it. As social creatures, we thrive when we share experiences, goals, and stories.

Finding Like-Minded Communities

Meetups & Clubs: Search "sober hike groups," "outdoor clubs," or anything that piques your interest.

Volunteer Organizations: Shelters, community gardens, youth mentorship. Helping others fosters empathy and belonging.

Online Spaces: If local options are slim, join digital communities for your hobby or for sober living support.

Loneliness as a Relapse Trigger

Isolation is one of the most overlooked threats to recovery. When you feel disconnected, it's easy for old cravings to creep back in—especially during moments of stress or emotional fatigue. But connection is more than just comfort—it's protection.

Studies have consistently shown that strong social support reduces the risk of relapse and improves long-term recovery outcomes. In fact, research published in the *Journal of Substance Abuse Treatment* (Beattie & Longabaugh, 1999) found that individuals with positive family interactions and meaningful peer support were significantly more likely to maintain sobriety. Feeling seen, understood, and supported by others reinforces your progress and makes it easier to keep moving forward.

Sustainable Evolution

Think of the "new you" as someone who never stops learning or striving. Even after you've built a stable foundation, keep exploring:

- **Continuous Learning:** Challenge yourself with new languages, instruments, or advanced certifications in your profession.

- **Mastery & Mentorship:** Once you become comfortable with a hobby (say, painting or yoga), consider teaching beginners or volunteering at workshops. Mentoring deepens your skill and sense of purpose.

- **Social Creativity:** Collaborate with friends on big projects—like forming a band, co-authoring a blog, or organizing a local event.

Momhak Moment

Sobriety isn't the final checkpoint. It's a new beginning to keep reinventing yourself, project after project, dream after dream.

Action Step

1. **Pick One Skill or Topic:** Something you've always admired or found intriguing—like learning to play the piano, starting a YouTube channel, or fixing a bicycle.

2. **Map a 30-Day Plan - Break It Down:** "Week 1: basic tutorials. Week 2: simple practice. Week 3: attempt a small challenge. Week 4: show or share it with a friend."

3. **Celebrate:** Each small milestone you reach is a testament to your capacity to learn and grow beyond addiction's confines.

Thriving, Not Just Surviving

Replace the Old Cravings

Overcoming addiction involves dismantling old pathways in the brain's reward circuitry. But as Dr. Lembke emphasizes, you can't just tear something down; you need to build something better in its place. Passion, community, creativity, and movement all become your new neural highways—routes that lead to genuine satisfaction rather than self-destruction.

If you remove a weed from a garden and leave the soil bare, more weeds may pop up. Planting flowers (new interests, new goals) ensures that you fill that space with beauty and growth.

Science Corner

As mentioned earlier, psychologist Mihaly Csikszentmihalyi's work on flow states—those immersive periods of deep focus and enjoyment—offers a powerful alternative to the artificial highs of addiction. By engaging in challenging, purposeful activities that fully absorb your attention, you activate the brain's natural reward system in a sustainable way. Replacing destructive dopamine spikes with the "clean high" of flow can fulfill your need for stimulation and mastery—all while significantly lowering the risk of relapse.

Personal Reflection

Sometimes I barely recognize the person who struggled to face each day without a drink. My mornings are now anchored in habits that feel second-nature: energizing breathwork combined with affirmations, and mindful movement that grounds me in clarity and strength. Yet these practices aren't the true measure of my transformation—they're just tools. The real shift is internal—it's the optimism, purpose, and peace I carry through each day, feelings I never believed possible during my darkest times. Today, addiction doesn't define me—I'm defined by curiosity, adventure, and a deep desire to share what I've learned. Writing this book is my way of offering you that same hope, affirming that together we can create lives filled not just with sobriety, but with true freedom, meaning, and joy.

"What lies behind us and what lies before us are tiny matters compared to what lies within us."
—Ralph Waldo Emerson

Once Addicted, Now Thriving

From Partygoer to Passionate Explorer

Previously caught up in endless nights at bars, they now redirect their resources and energy into adventures, exploring national parks and distant cultures abroad. Each new destination becomes a celebration of freedom, discovery, and genuine joy.

From Binge Drinker to Empowered Athlete

Transforming their former compulsions into dedication, they now channel intense focus into marathon training. Every race completed isn't just a physical achievement but a powerful affirmation of newfound strength and self-worth.

From Isolation to Community Inspiration

Previously withdrawn and consumed by addiction at home, they now step boldly into their community, volunteering and eventually taking leadership roles. Through service and connection, they discover profound meaning, resilience, and a deep sense of belonging.

Momhak Moment

Recovery is about rediscovering parts of yourself that addiction smothered—and then lighting them up so brightly that old habits have no room to re-enter.

Practical Steps to Design Your Future

Putting all of this into action can feel daunting. Here's a blueprint to get you started:

1. Passion Snapshot (Deep Dive Edition): Uncover what truly lights you up and begin building a life around it.

Free-Write First: Set a timer for 5 to 10 minutes and list anything that excites you—travel, fitness, art, cooking, animals, activism, nature, writing, science, music, teaching, or something you've always been curious about. No filter.

Spot the Sparks: Circle 2 or 3 passions that give you an energy jolt just thinking about them.

Take the First Step: For each circled passion, write down one tangible action.
Example: "For music, I'll dust off my guitar and practice 15 minutes each morning," or "For animals, I'll volunteer once a week at the local shelter."

2. Movement Integration Plan: Make movement a cornerstone of your new lifestyle—and a source of clean dopamine.

Set a Weekly Rhythm: Aim for at least three movement sessions (walks, dance, swimming, Qi Gong, weightlifting, martial arts—whatever suits you). Pick days and times that are realistic.

Make It Social: Invite a friend, join a class, or track your progress with others online using **#Momhak365**.

Notice the Shift: Journal or reflect on how you feel before and after each session. You'll start to see the power of movement in real time—better mood, better sleep, better mindset.

3. Purpose Alignment Ritual: Infuse your daily life with your deeper values—your "Why."

Morning Intention: Ask, *Does today reflect the kind of person I'm becoming?* Let this guide how you spend your time and energy.

Evening Reflection: Before bed, ask, *Did I live in alignment with my purpose today?* If not, identify one simple shift for tomorrow. This daily check-in keeps your compass pointed toward the life you're building.

4. Build Your Tribe: Transformation is personal—but thriving happens in connection.

Find Your People: Search for local meetups, online forums, classes, or sober-living communities connected to your interests—and also connect online with fellow Momhak Method practitioners via the website resources or **#Momhak365**.

Keep Showing Up: It's okay to feel awkward or out of place at first. Consistency builds connection.

Give What You Want to Get: Celebrate someone else's win. Offer support. Encourage newcomers. Community is a mirror—what you put in comes back to you tenfold.

5. Lifestyle Upgrades That Stick: Your energy, time, and money are now powerful tools—use them to elevate your life.

Invest in Experience: Channel your freed-up funds into something that feeds your soul—like weekend getaways, outdoor gear, dance lessons, or wellness workshops.

Keep Learning: Take a free course, attend a public lecture, or try a new skill through YouTube, Skillshare, or your local library. Growth is the antidote to stagnation.

Become a Mentor: When you're ready, help someone who's just starting out. Share your story. Teach a tool. Leading others deepens your own growth and rewires your identity as someone who uplifts.

Final Summary: Thriving Beyond Sobriety

Core Message

Sobriety isn't the end goal—it's the fertile ground on which to cultivate a life so fulfilling that you naturally choose growth over relapse. By actively designing your days—infusing them with passions, movement, purpose, and community support—you transform recovery from a defensive stance into a joyful, forward-looking journey.

Key Lessons

Fill Your Days with Life-Affirming Activities: Turn your old "substance time" into creative or social pursuits that expand your skill set and relationships.

Movement as a Cornerstone: Consistent exercise fosters well-being, resilience, and stable dopamine.

Align with Your "Why": Continually anchor daily routines in your deeper mission. This merges external actions with internal values, strengthening your resolve.

Build Your Tribe: Seek out those who champion your evolution. Loneliness can be a hidden relapse trigger; community is the antidote.

Keep Evolving: Master new skills, push your boundaries, and share your knowledge with others. Growth wards off stagnation and keeps your mind engaged.

Quick Win: Create A Passion Snapshot

1. Write down three things that make you feel truly alive—whether it's painting, dancing, or volunteering.

2. Schedule one for this week, even if it's only 10 minutes.

3. Reflect: Did you feel more energized, curious, or proud? Embrace that spark.

Your #Momhak365 Challenge: Design Your Future

Over the next 7 days:

- **Identify Passions**: Revisit your old loves or test new interests

- **Commit to Movement**: Incorporate some form of exercise or physical activity regularly

- **Engage Creatively**: Art, music, writing, or tinkering fosters healthy dopamine loops

- **Surround Yourself with Growth**: Whether it's a local group or online forum, connect with others on a similar upward trajectory

- **Track the Changes**: Journal how your energy, mood, and sense of purpose shift

Bonus: Share a snippet of your new hobby or plan using **#Momhak365**. You might inspire someone else to try an art class or sign up for a 5K race.

Mindful Moment: Envision Your Future

1. Close Your Eyes: Inhale for 4 seconds, exhale for 6.

2. Imagine: Picture the next year of your life, lived with clarity, purpose, and a schedule brimming with meaningful pursuits.

3. See: Envision the people you meet, the skills you develop, the confidence that grows day by day.

4. **Feel:** Wrap yourself in an undercurrent of gratitude, knowing that you broke free from addiction's loop and stepped into creative, expansive living.

Looking Ahead: Your Journey Continues

Even though this is the final chapter of the book, your real-life transformation keeps going. You now have the strategies to:

- **Refine & Expand Your Purpose**: As you grow, your values may shift. That's normal. Embrace it.

- **Solidify Habits**: Keep returning to the Four Pillars of The Momhak Method (Cold Exposure, Mindful Breathing, Moving Meditation, Mind Hacking).

- **Share Your Story**: Whether through online posts, local groups, or personal conversations, your insights can light a path for someone else in darkness.

This is your new life: an ongoing series of milestones, each fueled by curiosity, hope, and a commitment to living fully.

Momhak Moment

You never "finish" thriving. It's a process of continuous renewal—day after day, choice after choice, breath after breath.

Remember: The story you write from here is yours. Yes, you overcame something huge—but that's merely a prologue to the life you're now creating. By dedicating yourself to purpose, movement, curiosity, and connection, you leave little room for relapse and every possibility for joy. You're no longer just surviving—you're thriving. **Embrace it**.

FINAL THOUGHTS: A LIFE BEYOND LIMITS

"The secret of change is to focus all of your energy, not on fighting the old, but on building the new."
—Socrates

You made it.

Not just to the end of this book but also to the beginning of a new story—a story in which you're no longer defined by what you've escaped from but by what you're stepping into.

Whether you're on Day 1 or Day 1,000 of sobriety, this moment is a threshold. You've reclaimed your time, your attention, your breath, and your body. And now comes the most exciting—and sometimes the most daunting—part of the journey: deciding what kind of life you want to build with that freedom.

This isn't a return to who you were before addiction. This is about becoming someone even stronger, clearer, and more connected. Someone with a calm mind, a resilient body, and a purpose that pulls you forward.

Who You Were… & Who You Are Now

Remember the version of you that picked up this book?

Maybe you were tired. Worn out. Maybe you were desperate for relief. Or perhaps you were simply curious—about whether change was possible, or about whether you were ready for it.

Maybe you didn't believe you had the discipline. Maybe you didn't even know where to start.

And yet, here you are.

You've learned how cravings are wired into your brain—and how they can be unwired. You've discovered how breath, cold, movement, and mindset aren't just tools for recovery—they're pathways to your power.

You've practiced showing up for yourself. Not perfectly, but consistently. And that's what creates momentum. That's what builds mastery.

You've Only Just Begun

A new identity is forming. Not as someone barely hanging on—but as someone learning to thrive. Maybe you've started a movement practice that you love. Maybe you're experimenting with Cold Exposure, journaling, joining a community, or setting boundaries for the first time in years.

Whatever path you've begun to carve, know this: **You're no longer who you were**. And that's worth celebrating.

But we also need to acknowledge something deeper.

The Grief That Comes with Growth

When you let go of addiction, you're also letting go of something that was once your coping mechanism, your escape, even your identity.

And there's grief in that.

There's grief in realizing how much time was lost.

There's grief in seeing what your brother, your sister, your friend—or your younger self—didn't get to experience.

But grief is not the enemy. Grief is a doorway. It means you're alive, awake, and capable of feeling again. And that, more than anything, is what allows joy to return.

Joy doesn't replace grief. It emerges **through it**.

So don't run from what hurts. Instead, let it remind you of what *matters*. Let it remind you of why you're doing this work.

The Core Promise of the Momhak Method

The Momhak Method doesn't ask you to be perfect. It asks you to participate.

It's not about mastering every tool on Day One. It's about beginning—taking small, consistent steps that generate momentum. You don't need to memorize the Four Pillars. You've already lived them: the moment you chose breath over panic, movement over numbness, and truth over denial, you stepped right into the method. It's not a checklist. It's a rhythm. A lifestyle.

What makes The Momhak Method different isn't just the tools. It's the mindset behind them. You're not broken. You're not powerless. You're not here to merely "quit." You're here to reclaim.

That's the real promise.

You don't have to fight your way forward. You get to build your way free.

This isn't about escape. It's about expansion.

Every affirmation, every cold rinse, every breath, every mindful step—that's not recovery. That's creation. That's you becoming who you're meant to be.

What You've Built

You didn't just read this book—you rewrote your story.

Each chapter was a doorway. And with every step, you moved closer to clarity, strength, and the version of yourself you were always meant to become.

Chapter 1: When Everything Changed

You began with a moment of reckoning—a low point, a wake-up call, or perhaps a quiet realization that something needed to shift. Rather than seeing your pain as punishment, you reframed it as a portal. A call to rise.

Chapter 2: Understanding the Wiring

You dove beneath the surface, learning how addiction alters brain chemistry and hijacks your reward system. Most importantly, you discovered that change isn't about brute force—it's about rewiring your brain through neuroplasticity and reclaiming your dopamine system naturally.

Chapter 3: Your First Step into the Method

You met the Four Pillars—Mind Hacking, Cold Exposure, Mindful Breathing, and Moving Meditation. Instead of a rigid program, you were given a flexible set of tools and encouraged to begin simply, letting consistency do the heavy lifting.

Chapter 4: Resetting the Body

You learned to disrupt stress patterns and reset your nervous system using cold, breath, and physical activation. This was about waking up the body—flushing out old tension and reintroducing clarity, energy, and calm.

Chapter 5: Movement as Medicine

You discovered that movement doesn't just burn calories—it heals. Through yoga, Tai Chi, Qi Gong, and other mindful movement, you found presence in motion and began syncing breath with body. Perfect for those who struggle with stillness, this was meditation you could feel.

Chapter 6: Mastering Your Inner Voice

You learned to speak to yourself differently. Using tools like CBT, affirmations, and the Pain–Pleasure Principle, you began replacing loops of self-sabotage with loops of self-leadership. Your thoughts no longer controlled you—you learned to shape them.

Chapter 7: Creating Daily Momentum

In this chapter, you built your lifestyle foundation. Morning rituals, breathwork, food choices, sleep hygiene—small, stacked habits that quietly recalibrate your entire identity over time. You stopped living in reaction and started living by design.

Chapter 8: Navigating the Social World

You learned to face the outside world on your own terms. With tools for boundary-setting, refusing drinks, and handling awkward conversations, you realized that sobriety doesn't mean isolation—it means finding relationships that respect your growth.

Chapter 9: Rediscovering Purpose

No longer defined by what you quit you began focusing on what you're here to **create**. You crafted your "Why," clarified your values, and glimpsed a future powered not by avoidance—but by *meaning*.

Chapter 10: Stepping Into Your Next Identity

You took your energy and time—the very things addiction once consumed—and redirected them toward passions, people, and purpose. You began building not just a sober life but a *thriving* one—anchored in movement, community, learning, and growth.

Living the Ongoing Transformation

Transformation isn't a one-time event; it's an unfolding journey. You'll encounter hurdles—stressful events, social triggers, and moments of old temptation. Instead of viewing these setbacks as failures, see them as checkpoints that help you recalibrate. Each challenge becomes a chance to recall why you started, and to prove how far you've come.

1. **Celebrate Your Wins:** Did you successfully handle an awkward social invitation? Did you take a 2-minute cold shower on a tough morning? Each small victory is tangible evidence of your growing strength.

2. **Refine Your "Why":** Perhaps your initial driver was to avoid hangovers. Now, maybe you're driven by a creative passion

you've recently rediscovered, or the desire to be fully present for loved ones.

3. **Check In Regularly:** Revisit your 5-month/5-year vision. You might be closer than you think, or you may have discovered an entirely new dream along the way.

Where You're Headed: Your 5-Year Vision

Close your eyes and imagine this: It's 5 years from now. You wake up energized. Your body feels strong. Your mind is clear. You've built a life full of purpose, movement, and connection. You've created something that matters.

You look back and realize that this moment—**where you are right now**—was the turning point.

That's the future you're building every time you choose movement over numbness.

Every time you choose breath over panic.

Every time you speak to yourself with kindness instead of cruelty.

Every time you remember who you're becoming.

It's OK to Be Not OK—Even Now

Even after all these chapters and breakthroughs, you'll still have off days. Don't interpret them as failure; they're part of the lifelong journey. Tough feelings and dips in motivation can reappear well beyond the "honeymoon" phase of sobriety. **Remember: you're not failing, and what you're feeling is normal.** Recall the tools you've gathered—breathwork, affirmations, mindful movement, a supportive community—and trust in your capacity to navigate these ups and downs with self-compassion.

Momhak Moment

Off days don't erase your progress—they remind you that you're human and that you have effective ways to handle life's ebbs and flows.

In other words, you've come too far to let an occasional rough patch define you. Keep the bigger picture in mind, honor your feelings, and remember that you have the skills to move through them.

Building Momentum & Support

You're Never Alone

Recovery flourishes in community. While self-reliance builds resilience, isolation can rekindle old fears or triggers. Seek or create your tribe by:

- **Joining Groups**: Whether it's a local hiking club, a sober group meet-up, or an online forum, connecting with others provides motivation and perspective.

- **Volunteering & Mentoring**: Nothing cements your new habits faster than guiding someone else. In helping them, you reinforce your own progress.

Personalizing the Momhak Method

Feel free to adapt each pillar—Mind Hacking, Cold Exposure, Mindful Breathing, Moving Meditation—to your own style. Some embrace ice baths. Others are content with a brisk cold shower. Some love yoga flows. Others prefer a daily run or lifting weights. The goal is to keep them consistent, enjoyable, and attuned to your needs.

Key Principles

Consistency: The best method is the one you can sustain.

Joy: If you dread an activity, tweak it until it feels rewarding or at least worthwhile.

Try It. Feel It. Make It Yours.

Now that you've explored each pillar of The Momhak Method, the next step is simple: Begin blending them into a rhythm that fits your life.

You don't need a perfect routine. You don't need to follow rigid steps. What matters is momentum—trying, observing, adjusting. Choose a few core practices you enjoy and begin weaving them into your mornings, your breaks, and your evenings.

Trust the method, but also trust yourself.

Whether it's Cold Exposure, Mindful Breathing, Moving Meditation, or Mind Hacking—when these tools are used together, they create synergy. A small, consistent daily practice can change your emotional baseline, build resilience, and create a powerful sense of forward motion.

And when you notice even the smallest shift—more calm, less stress, deeper clarity—celebrate it. Let those moments remind you: **you're doing it**. You're changing.

Share the Shift with #Momhak365

You don't have to do this alone. When you share your progress, even privately with a friend or journaling app, you reinforce your transformation. And when you speak it out loud—to a community, online, or to someone just starting their journey—you might be the spark that changes another life.

This is how movements grow.

A Life Beyond Limits

The Momhak Method is more than a path to sobriety—it's a blueprint for personal evolution. Each practice you've explored isn't just about breaking free from addiction; it's about building something extraordinary in its place. This is your invitation to keep going—not in struggle but in growth. Not in fear but in curiosity. Not just sober—but **alive**.

Let your life expand. Explore movement, hobbies, and creative passions that light you up. Whether it's surfing, hiking, dancing, or painting—immerse yourself in activities that nourish your body and awaken your joy. These aren't distractions from the work—they *are* the work. They rewire your brain, stabilize your mood, and reconnect you to your true self.

Stay mindful. Keep breathing deeply. Stay curious about new ways to ground your nervous system and expand your awareness. Whether through seated meditation, Qi Gong, or a walking practice, presence is the thread that holds it all together.

Revisit your affirmations. Let them anchor you on days when motivation runs low. These simple phrases aren't fluff—they're tools that reshape your inner dialogue and hardwire self-respect into your identity.

And above all, lead with gratitude and compassion. Gratitude turns the ordinary into a gift. Compassion allows you to keep moving even when you stumble. This journey isn't about perfection—it's about progress, patience, and presence.

And finally, when you're ready, pay it forward. Share what's worked for you. Tell your story. Mentor someone who's just starting out. Every time you help someone else rise, you rise as well. This is how recovery becomes a ripple effect—turning your transformation into someone else's permission slip.

You've come this far. And the life ahead of you? It's not just worth staying sober for—it's worth celebrating, exploring, and expanding into fully.

Final Thoughts Takeaway

The Momhak Method is more than a set of tactics—it's a framework for living fully. Each chapter introduced tools—cold showers, meditations, cognitive reframing, purposeful daily habits—that become most powerful when layered consistently.

Think of them as instruments in an orchestra, generating harmony for your mental, physical, and spiritual well-being.

Take Heart

You've already proven your capacity for change simply by reaching this point. A world brimming with adventure, creativity, and meaningful connections awaits. Continue layering habits, anchoring to your core values, and trusting that each mindful day carries you closer to the thriving life you deserve.

Remember that the journey doesn't end at sobriety. It begins with the freedom to design a life on your own terms.

What You've Gained

Along the way, you've gained far more than just sobriety.

You've gained **momentum**—the kind that compounds with each breath, each habit, each conscious choice. Every time you showed up for yourself, you weren't just staying sober—you were actively rewiring your brain for long-term success and resilience.

You've found **connection**. Whether through shared experiences, new communities, or simply realizing you're not alone, you now stand beside a growing circle of others committed to living with intention and freedom. Sobriety isn't isolation—it's a doorway into deeper belonging.

And maybe most powerfully, you've found **evidence**. Proof that growth is possible. That healing is real. That even one month, six months, or one year from now, your life can be utterly transformed by the quiet power of small, consistent steps.

You've done more than survive.

You've proven that you can *thrive*.

Final Momhak Moment

Small, consistent choices shape a remarkable destiny. You don't need perfection—just the resolve to show up for yourself, day after day, breath by breath.

A Challenge & An Invitation

You've done the inner work. Now go live it.

Take a cold shower and scream with joy. Breathe into the discomfort and feel your power. Walk into the world with your head high and your nervous system calm. Say "no" when you need to. Say "yes" to what excites you. Be weird. Be wild. Be wonderfully, fully *you*.

And if you ever feel lost again, remember this:

You have the tools.

You have the body.

You have the breath.

You have the method.

Now go make a life you're proud of.

***

My life changed for the better in every possible way since becoming sober. I wish the same for you—and for anyone you may inspire on your journey. It's a cliché, yes, but it's true: What doesn't kill you makes you stronger. Always keep that in mind when thinking of your own trials and tribulations. I hope that the reflections, stories, and techniques in this book help you break free and find genuine joy.

I love being sober—there's no other feeling like it in the world. I hope you find the same enjoyment in sobriety that I have, and that I wish my brother could've found as well.

APPENDIX A: ESSENTIAL EXERCISES FROM THE MOMHAK METHOD

A structured roadmap of key exercises from The Momhak Method, organized by chapter and phase.

PHASE 1: Understanding & Resetting Your Brain
(Introduction and Chapters 1–3)

Introduction

Create Your Personal Power Affirmation

Your thoughts shape your reality, so let's build a foundation. You'll use a **Personal Power Affirmation** as a mental anchor—your quick go-to for motivation, focus, or a reset.

How to Create Yours:

- **Positive**: Focus on what you want, not what you're avoiding.

- **Present-Tense**: "I am strong" rather than "I will be strong."

- **Personal**: It should resonate with your unique goals.

Examples:

- "I'm strong, clear-headed, and in control."

- "I'm calm and focused, thriving in sobriety."

- "Every day, I'm creating a life I love."

Write it down, say it aloud, place it somewhere visible. And remember: Your affirmations aren't set in stone; they should evolve alongside your growth and changing needs. What empowers you today may transform as *you* transform, so revisit and refresh your personal power statements as your journey unfolds.

Two Possible Futures Visualization

This exercise—visualizing two possible futures—was introduced to me in *The 30-Day Sobriety Solution* (Andrews & Canfield, 2016), and it's one I've returned to many times.

1. Find a Quiet Spot: Have a journal or device handy.

2. Center Yourself: Take 3 slow breaths: Inhale deeply for 4 counts, then exhale slowly for 6 counts.

3. Embrace Honesty: This is about clarity, not blame or shame.

Part 1: The Path of Continued Struggle

1. Envision Yourself 5 Months from Now If Nothing Changes

- How might your health worsen?

- Which relationships could deteriorate or end?

- How might finances, career, or daily mood suffer?

2. Envision Yourself 5 Years from Now If Nothing Changes

- Any irreversible damage to your health?

- Which dreams or opportunities might be lost?

- Does it echo my brother's fate?

These questions aren't to scare you but rather to highlight where you could find yourself if you remain stuck.

Part 2: The Path of Transformation

1. Envision Yourself 5 Months from Now Embracing The Momhak Method

- How could your energy, sleep, and overall health improve?

- Which habits or skills might make you proud?

- How does each morning feel when you wake up?

- Which friendships or family relationships start to heal or grow stronger?

2. Envision Yourself 5 Years from Now Embracing The Momhak Method

- How might your mind and body flourish?

- Which achievements excite you most?

- How do your closest relationships evolve?

- Which passions have you rekindled or newly discovered?

- How might your financial situation have improved, providing greater security and freedom?

- How does it feel to be **fully alive** in your own life?

Chapter 1: The Moment Everything Changed

The "Moment of Truth" Reflection

- Write down the hardest truth you've faced about your habit.

- Reflect: What was the wake-up call that made you realize you needed change?

- Action Step: Identify a single shift you can make today toward a different future.

Breathwork for Emotional Reset

- Inhale for 4 seconds, exhale for 6.

- Practice this when facing emotional distress or cravings.

Two-Paths Visualization Revisit

- Close your eyes. Imagine your life 5 years from now if you continue as you are.

- Now imagine it 5 years from now if you commit to change.

- Write down what excites you about the second vision.

Small First-Step Commitment

- Choose one action to take today toward change.
- Examples: Tell a friend, write a journal entry, or drink a glass of water instead of a beer.

Chapter 2: The Science of Addiction & Change

Dopamine Awareness Audit

- List all artificial dopamine sources in your life (alcohol, social media, junk food, etc.).
- Observe when and why you use them.
- Identify at least one **natural dopamine** alternative (exercise, deep breathing, music, cold exposure).

Decode Your Triggers

- Think of the last time you drank (or indulged in any habit you want to break).
- Identify the trigger (stress, boredom, loneliness, celebration?).
- Ask, *What was I hoping to get—relief, escape, excitement?*
- Now find a **healthier alternative** that delivers the same feeling minus the crash.

Reprogramming Your Reward System

- Close your eyes. Inhale for 4, then exhale for 6.
- Envision your brain as a series of paths in a dense forest.
- Each drink or destructive habit deepens the worn trail.
- Each healthy choice forges a new path.
- Ask yourself, *Which new trail am I deepening or creating today?*

Chapter 3: QuickStart to The Momhak Method

The 24-Hour Dopamine Detox

- Identify your biggest dopamine triggers (alcohol, excessive phone use, sugar etc.).

- Replace them for 24 to 48 hours with **clean dopamine** sources (walk in nature, cold shower, deep conversation).

- Journal any differences in mood or cravings.

Mind Hacking – Affirmation Integration

Pair your Personal Power Affirmation with a daily activity (saying it during a walk, brushing your teeth, while showering, etc.).

Diaphragmatic Breathing

- Sit or lie down in a relaxed position. Place one hand on your chest and one hand on your belly.

- Breathe in slowly for 4 to 6 seconds, allowing your belly to expand. The hand on your chest should remain still while the hand on your belly rises.

- Let the breath out gently for 6 to 8 seconds, feeling your belly fall.

- Repeat for 5 to 10 minutes: Focus on slow, controlled breaths, ensuring that your belly, not your chest, is moving.

PHASE 2: Physical & Mental Reset
(Chapters 4–6)

Chapter 4: The Physical Reset (Cold Exposure & Breathwork)

4–6 Breathing

How: Inhale through your nose for a count of 4, then exhale for 6.

Why: The prolonged extended exhale activates the parasympathetic nervous system, lowering stress hormones like cortisol and shifting you from fight-or-flight to rest-and-digest (Brown & Gerbarg, 2009).

When: Perfect for quick stress relief—traffic jams, mini-breaks, or pre-sleep calm.

4–7–8 Breathing

How: Inhale through your nose for 4 seconds, hold for 7, then exhale for 8.

Why: This technique can swiftly reduce anxiety, making it a favorite among insomniacs seeking calm before bed. By increasing the exhale time and adding a breath-hold, you deepen the relaxation effect.

Contraindications: If extended breath holds feel uncomfortable, shorten the hold time. Always listen to your body's cues.

Tummo/Wim Hof Breathing

Origins: A Tibetan Buddhist practice popularized by Dutch motivational speaker Wim Hof.

How:

- Lie down in a safe environment (never while driving or immersed in water).

- Take 30 deep, rhythmic breaths—fully inhaling and letting each exhale flow naturally.

- After the last breath, exhale about 90% and hold until you feel discomfort.

- Inhale fully, hold for 10 to 15 seconds, then release.

230

- Repeat for 3 rounds.

Why:

- **Boosts Immune Response:** In one clinical trial, participants using Wim Hof breathing plus cold exposure showed reduced inflammatory markers when exposed to an endotoxin (Kox et al., 2014).

- **Stress Adaptation:** Regulates the body's response to external stressors, teaching the mind to stay calm in high-stress situations.

- **Energy & Focus:** Tummo breathing can lead to a "clean" surge of energy, clarity, and potentially higher oxygen saturation.

- **Mood Lift:** Many practitioners—including myself—report a noticeable elevation in mood for hours after a session.

Safety: If you feel dizzy or faint, stop. Never combine breath holds with driving or swimming.

Weekly Schedule & Tracking

Consistency cements these new habits. Here's a **7-day plan** to incrementally scale Cold Exposure and Mindful Breathing. Feel free to modify.

Day	Cold Exposure	Breathing Practice	Notes/Journal
1	15-second cold shower	5 rounds of 4–6 breathing (morning)	Post-shower mood/energy
2	20-second cold shower	1 or 2 of rounds Tummo/Wim Hof; use affirmations during breath holds	Track your breath holds. Which felt easiest?
3	25-second cold shower	4–7–8 breathing before bed (5 rounds)	Rate your sleep quality the next morning

4	30-second cold shower	2 or 3 Tummo rounds daily; affirmations during breath holds	Any emotional shifts? More or fewer cravings?
5	35-second cold shower	5 rounds 4–6 midday or under stress	Observe dips in your energy or stress
6	40-second cold shower	3 Tummo rounds (morning) + 4–7–8 (night)	Compare morning vs. night mental states
7	40- to 60-second cold shower	Choose any combo of technique + affirmations	Evaluate. Which approach resonates most?

Reflection: Note changes in your mood, cravings, energy, and sleep. This loop helps you spot what's most beneficial.

Expanded Monthly Progression Plan

If you want more than a 7-day schedule, try this **4-week** progression:

Week	Cold Exposure	Breathing Practice	Focus
1	10- to 30-second cold shower, 3x/week	2 or 3 Tummo + affirmations daily	Get comfortable with basics
2	30- to 60-second cold shower, 4 or5x/week	2 or 3 Tummo + affirmations daily, 4–7–8 breathing at night	Notice calmer evenings and stable mood
3	60- to 120-second cold shower, nearly daily	2 or 3 Tummo + affirmations daily, 4–6 breathing when stressed	Amplify dopamine boost; track emotional balance
4	60- to 120-second cold shower, daily;	3 Tummo + affirmations daily, 4–6 breathing at bedtime	Solidify routine; refine best techniques

	optional cold plunge		

Tracking: Each Sunday, review your notes. Are certain breath exercises more helpful during cravings? Does your overall stress or sleep improve?

Chapter 5: Moving Meditation

Emergency 2-Minute Stress Craving Intervention

When stress or cravings strike, try this **movement-based sequence** in under 2 minutes. Craft an affirmation made of two lines: one that fits the rhythm of a 4-second inhale, and one that fits the rhythm of a 6-second exhale. Let the words match your breath. Stand or sit with your feet firmly grounded. Let your arms hang relaxed at your sides. Begin a simple flowing movement:

- Inhale slowly for 4 seconds as you slowly lift your arms up in front of you, palms facing forward and fingers pointing inward while you repeat your 4-second affirmation.

- Exhale slowly for 6 seconds as you lower your arms down in a circular motion along your sides, palms facing outward and fingers pointing up while you repeat your 6-second affirmation.

Repeat this breath-movement-affirmation cycle 6 times, letting your motion follow the rhythm of your breath.
Final Shift: Walk in place or do a gentle stretch for 30 seconds, bridging mind and body so that stress can't take hold.

The Tai Chi Walk

1. Start in a Relaxed, Centered Stance

- Stand with feet hip to shoulder-width apart, knees slightly bent.

- Keep your spine straight, shoulders relaxed, and gaze forward.

- Place your hands gently at your sides.

2. Shift Your Weight & Step Forward

- Slowly shift your weight onto your right foot as you inhale deeply through the nose.

- Lift your left foot just off the ground, keeping it relaxed.

- Extend the left foot forward and place the heel down first while keeping most of your weight on the back leg.

3. Transfer Weight Gradually

- As you **exhale slowly through the mouth,** begin shifting your weight forward onto the left foot.

- Feel the smooth transition as your back foot becomes lighter.

- Once fully balanced on the left foot, **lift the right foot off the ground** for the next step.

4. Repeat the Process

- Continue moving forward at a slow, controlled pace, fully shifting weight before lifting the back foot.

- Maintain deep, rhythmic breathing—inhale as you lift and step, exhale as you shift and root.

- Stay relaxed, keeping movements fluid, soft, and intentional.

5. Maintain Awareness

- Focus on each movement, each breath, and each point of contact with the ground.

- Imagine gliding forward smoothly, as if moving through water.

- Keep your mind calm and present, fully engaged in the act of walking.

Microcosmic Orbit Flow with Arm Movements

This exercise combines **breathwork, visualization,** and **flowing arm movements** to enhance relaxation and energy circulation through the body.

How to Practice:

1. Start in a Standing Position

- Stand with feet hip-width apart, knees slightly bent, back strait, chin tucked.

- Relax your shoulders and do a few rounds of abdominal/diaphragmatic breathing, paying more attention to the exhalations than the inhalations. Gently press the tip of your tongue on the palate of your mouth.

2. Inhale – Arms Rise – Energy Moves Up the Spine

- As you **inhale**, raise your arms slowly up your sides, keeping them straight with your palms facing down and your fingers together.

- Imagine energy rising from the base of the spine (Huiyin point) up along your **back to the crown of your head**.

- Keep the move smooth and continuous, ending with your arms lifted to shoulder or head height.

3. Exhale – Arms Lower – Energy Moves Down the Front Centerline

- As your inhale peaks, begin your exhale and bring your hands together in front of your face with your palms facing inward.

- Continue the **exhale slowly** as your **hands move down the front of your body**, tracing a path from your face to your lower abdomen.

- Visualize energy flowing **down the front of your body**, from the crown of your head to just below the navel.

4. Repeat & Flow

- Continue this movement for **5 to 10 minutes**, synchronizing your breath with the movement.

- Feel the energy circulating smoothly: rising up the spine, over the crown of the head, descending down the front of the body, and returning to the lower abdomen.

5. Complete the Cycle – Return to Center

- To end the exercise, bring your hands gently to rest over your lower abdomen, one hand placed on top of the other. Let your palms softly cradle your belly, with your thumbs touching, forming a small hollow where your belly button sits nestled between them. This position helps you anchor attention in the body's energetic center, located just below the navel.

- Take a few rounds of slow, diaphragmatic breathing, allowing your abdomen to rise and fall naturally beneath your hands. With each breath, feel your energy gathering and consolidating in your core.

- This is your return point—your center. End your practice with calm awareness and gratitude for the energy you've cultivated.

- To finish, rub your hands briskly together then massage your face, head, ears and neck.

Chapter 6: Mind Hacking – Rewiring Your Inner World

Pleasure–Pain Rewiring (Tony Robbins' NAC)

- Identify the habit you want to change.

- Associate massive pain with the old habit.

- Load the Pleasure of Change by training your brain to crave the rewards of your new path.

- Write 3 painful consequences of your old habit.

- Write 3 pleasurable rewards of quitting.

Craft a Pain-Pleasure Affirmation

1. **Select Your Habit:** For example—quitting alcohol or smoking, or even negative self-talk.

2. **Identify the Pain:** Write 3 bullet points describing the pain this habit brings you. Example: "I lose money, I lose respect, and I hurt my body."

3. **Identify the Pleasure:** Write 3 bullet points of the blessings you'll gain by stopping. Example: "I'll have more money, more energy, and more confidence."

4. **Formulate a One-Sentence Affirmation:** Combine both. For instance:

   "Alcohol poisons my health, relationships and happiness; thriving in sobriety brings me real joy, calmness, and success."

5. **Say It Daily:** Morning, before bed, and whenever a craving strikes.

Reframe Negative Thoughts

- Recognize automatic negative thoughts.

- Challenge them (Are they really true?).

- Replace with positive, empowering thoughts.

Forgiveness Practice

- Identify moments of regret.

- Say: "I did my best with what I knew. I release this guilt."

- Write down a list of past regrets, then write a compassionate reframe for each one—turning guilt into growth by acknowledging what you learned and how you've changed.

PHASE 3: Consistency, Confidence & Connection
(Chapters 7–8)

Chapter 7: Daily Habits for Thriving

Morning (30 to 45 minutes total)

1. Breathwork & Affirmations (10 minutes)

Tummo breathing with affirmations and mindfulness during breath holds. "I'm clear-headed and strong, thriving in sobriety."

2. Cold Shower (1 or 2 minutes)

Add a 30-second cold burst to your regular shower—either at the beginning, middle, or end.

3. Micro-Journal (5 minutes)

Note your top intention for the day: "Today, I prioritize calm and kindness."

Midday (2 to 5 minutes each break)

1. 1 minute of 4–6 breathing every time you feel stress spiking

2. Quick walk around the building or block

3. Healthy snack/hydration check

Evening (15 to 30 minutes)

1. Tech-Free Wind-Down Time (at least 30 minutes before bed)

Dim the lights, put away devices.

2. Gratitude Journal (5 minutes)

Note one win of the day, no matter how small.

3. Gentle Movement or Body Scan (5 to 10 minutes)

Yin yoga, mild stretching, or scanning from toes to head.

Nighttime Sleep (7 to 9 hours)

1. Keep your bedroom cool and dark

2. Maintain a regular bedtime

3. Avoid caffeine after 2 p.m.

Sustainability: Start small. If 45 minutes each morning sounds impossible, do 5 to 10 minutes. Let success breed success.

See Who You're Becoming

- Close your eyes. Take a deep breath in for 4 seconds, then exhale for 6.

- Imagine yourself 6 months from now, thriving in a life built on strong, daily habits.

- See yourself waking up refreshed, eating nourishing food, and handling stress with ease.

- Every small habit you build today is shaping this future version of you.

Chapter 8: Mastering Social Challenges

Create Your "No" Script

Prepare for social situations by practicing a simple, confident way to refuse a drink.

1. Choose a response that feels natural to you:

- **Polite but firm:** "I'm good with what I have, thanks."

- **Direct:** "I don't drink anymore—it's the best decision I've ever made."

- **Lighthearted:** "I've had enough drinks for a lifetime!"

2. Practice saying it out loud.

3. Visualize yourself using it in a real-life situation.

THC Decision Matrix

Question	High-Risk Answer	Potentially Safe Answer
Why am I using THC?	To escape or avoid my emotions.	To manage a legit medical condition.
How often do I use it?	Daily or multiple times a day.	Occasionally, with specific purpose.

How does it affect my progress?	Increases anxiety or apathy.	Reduces my cravings or helps me function.
Do I crave it when it's unavailable?	Yes, I get anxious or irritable.	No, I can easily take it or leave it.
Have I consulted a professional?	No, I'm winging it on my own.	Yes, I've spoken to a therapist/doctor.

- **If multiple answers are in the high-risk column**, you may be substituting one dependency for another.

- **If your usage is on the safer side**—sporadic, mindful, and guided by medical or therapeutic input—it might be a short-term tool.

PHASE 4: Purpose, Meaning & Long-Term Transformation
(Chapters 9–10)

Chapter 9: Finding Purpose & Meaning

Find Your Core Values
Follow these steps to uncover your core values:

1. **Reflect on Peak Moments:** Think of a time when you felt truly alive or deeply fulfilled. What value was being expressed in that moment (e.g., growth, connection, nature)?

2. **Notice Anger Triggers:** Often, we get most upset when a fundamental belief is violated. If dishonesty upsets you, honesty may be one of your core values.

3. **Write Down 3 to 5 Keywords:** From the list in Chapter 9, pick the values that resonate most with you. These will become the foundation for your "Why" Statement.

Creating Your "Why" Statement

Once you've chosen your core values, it's time to craft a personal "Why" Statement. A strong "Why" gives you direction and motivation, especially when cravings or self-doubt surface.

Example Formula:

"I live to [core value] by [action or behavior] so that I can [impact or outcome]."

Examples:

- "I live to experience life fully by embracing each moment with curiosity so that I can stay grounded in the now."

- "I live to strengthen my mind by choosing discipline over distraction so that I can reclaim my freedom."

- "I live to lead by example by walking the path of recovery so that I can show others that freedom is possible."

- "I live to cultivate resilience by staying active and facing challenges head-on so that I can live with strength and confidence."

- "I live to make a difference by sharing my story and tools so that I can help others heal and rise."

Action Steps:

1. Choose 3 to 5 core values from the list in Chapter 9.

2. Craft a single "Why" Statement based on those values.

3. Write it down and place it somewhere you'll see it daily (e.g., your mirror, phone screen, or journal).

Rewrite Your Identity

Think of one limiting label you've carried—maybe something like "I'm a screw-up," "I always relapse," or "I'm not strong enough." Now rewrite it into an empowering identity rooted in growth and possibility. Start with this format:

- **Old Label:** "I'm _____."

- **New Identity:** "I'm someone who _____."

Examples:
- **Old:** "I'm a failure."
  New: "I'm someone who learns from every challenge and keeps growing."

- **Old:** "I'm just an addict."
  New: "I'm a resilient person building a life I love."

Write it down. Say it out loud. Post it somewhere visible. This is how you begin living as your future self—today.

Ikigai (Japanese Concept of "Reason for Being")
Ikigai is often depicted as the overlap of four circles:

- What you love

- What you're good at

- What the world needs

- What can support you financially (or at least not harm your stability)

While you don't need to follow the model rigidly, exploring these categories can spark fresh insights:

- **What do I love doing?** Think of childhood passions or current curiosities.

- **What am I good at?** Could be professional skills or personal traits (e.g., empathy, organizing).

- **What does the world around me need?** A local cause? Mentorship? Creative expression that uplifts?

- **How do I ensure that I'm stable financially or practically?** This might mean adjusting a hobby into a side pursuit or a career pivot.

Practical Tip: Sketch out a 2 x 2 grid or overlapping circles. Brainstorm each corner. Even small intersections can reveal ways to live with more meaning.

Embracing Purpose Amid Imperfections

- **Close Your Eyes**: Inhale for 4 seconds, exhale for 6.

- **Visualize**: A scenario in which you woke up feeling "not OK." Picture yourself pausing, breathing, and choosing a purposeful act—maybe going for a walk or journaling about gratitude.

- **Notice**: How a small purposeful step transforms your mood. Let that calm or resolve spread through your body.

- **Accept**: The path isn't perfect; it's human. Emotions fluctuate, but your deeper mission remains.

Chapter 10: Thriving Beyond Sobriety

Reclaim Your Curiosity

- **Pick One Skill or Topic**: Something you've always admired or found intriguing—like learning to play the piano, writing a blog, or fixing a bicycle.

- **Map a 30-Day Plan - Break it Down**: "Week 1: basic tutorials. Week 2: simple practice. Week 3: attempt a small challenge. Week 4: show or share it with a friend."

- **Celebrate**: Each small milestone you reach is a testament to your capacity to learn and grow beyond addiction's confines.

Envision Your Future

- **Close Your Eyes**: Inhale for 4 seconds, exhale for 6.

- **Imagine**: The next year of your life, lived with clarity, purpose, and a schedule brimming with meaningful pursuits.

- **See**: The people you meet, the skills you develop, the confidence that grows day by day.

- **Feel**: An undercurrent of gratitude that you broke free from addiction's loop and stepped into creative, expansive living.

Final Notes

Each of these exercises builds toward rewiring the brain, fostering resilience, and creating a meaningful life beyond addiction. Whether you're just starting or deep into transformation, these tools provide a structured, actionable path.

For further support, visit **momhak.com.**

APPENDIX B: 30-DAY MOMHAK365 CHALLENGE

Welcome to the Momhak365 30-Day Challenge—a daily roadmap designed to help you reset your nervous system, rewire your habits, and rebuild your sense of purpose through small, consistent action.

Each day offers a structured practice involving cold exposure, breathwork, movement, and journaling or visualization. These suggestions are carefully aligned with the chapters in *The Momhak Method* and are meant to deepen your transformation—not overwhelm it.

That said, feel free to adapt the practices to fit your lifestyle. If you're already doing a different form of movement or breathwork, you can substitute accordingly. That said, I encourage you to try the recommended exercises at least once—even briefly—to stretch into unfamiliar terrain and discover new tools that might serve you.

Consistency matters, but so does curiosity. Treat each day as an experiment in presence, resilience, and self-leadership.

Day	Chapter	Cold Ex.	Breathing Practice	Moving Meditation Practice	Journaling / Visualizing
1	Intro	10- to 30-second cold shower	3 rounds 4–6 breathing	Mindful walk while repeating your Personal Power Affirmation	Create a present-tense, emotionally resonant Personal Power Affirmation

2	Intro	10- to 30-second cold shower	3 rounds 4–7–8 breathing	Mindful walk outside; be present in your breath and body as you walk	Envisioning two possible futures (one shaped by inaction, one by transformation); 5-Month and 5-Year Visualization
3	Chapter 1	10- to 30-second cold shower	5 rounds 4–6 breathing	Yin Yoga (gentle stretching) when you rise and before bed	Moment of Truth: Describe the turning point that made you want to change
4	Chapter 1	Optional cold shower	5 rounds 4–7–8 breathing	Mindful walk while repeating your Personal Power Affirmation	Revisit the Two-Paths Visualization: Compare your future in 5 months and 5 years if you continue as you are vs. if you commit to change

| 5 | Chapter 2 | 10- to 30-second cold shower | 2 or 3 rounds Tummo breathing + affirmations during breath holds | Yin Yoga (gentle stretching) when you rise and before bed | Mapping Emotional Cravings: Think of the last time you used. Identify 2 triggers (stress, boredom) and how they showed up |
| 6 | Chapter 2 | Optional cold shower | 2 or 3 rounds Tummo breathing + affirmations during breath holds + 4–7–8 breathing before bed | Mindful walk outside; be present in your breath and body as you walk | Dopamine Audit: List your top sources of artificial dopamine (e.g., alcohol, social media, junk food), then identify at least one natural alternative (e.g., exercise, music, cold exposure) |

| 7 | Chapter 3 | 10- to 30-second cold shower | 2 or 3 rounds Tummo breathing + affirmations and mindfulness during breath holds | Walk while repeating your Personal Power Affirmation aloud or silently, syncing it with your breath | Dopamine Detox: For the next 1 or 2 days, try cutting out your biggest artificial dopamine sources, replacing them with healthier dopamine-boosting activities; journal your results |
| 8 | Chapter 3 | 30- to 60-second cold shower | 2 or 3 rounds Tummo breathing + affirmations during breath holds | Diaphragmatic Breathing: Place one hand on your chest and one hand on your belly; practice 4–6 breathing; breathe for 5 to 10 minutes so that your belly moves and your chest stays still. | Revisit the Two-Paths Visualization (as above) |

9	Chapter 3	30- to 60-second cold shower	2 or 3 rounds Tummo breathing + affirmations during breath holds + 4–6 breathing before bed	Stand in place after your shower, breathe deeply, and scan your body from head to toe	After your cold shower, describe how your body and mind felt before and after the exposure
10	Chapter 4	30- 60-second cold shower	2 or 3 rounds Tummo breathing + affirmations during breath holds + 4–7–8 breathing before bed	Create and repeat an affirmation during your cold shower	In-Shower Focus Reflection: What affirmation did you use? How did it affect the cold shower experience?
11	Chapter 4	30- 60-second cold shower	2 or 3 rounds Tummo breathing + affirmations during breath holds	Mindful walk outside; be present in your breath and body as you walk	Journal how each technique (Tummo breathing, 4–6, 4–7–8) affects your mood and energy

12	Chapter 4	30- to 60-second cold shower	3 or 4 rounds Tummo breathing + affirmations during breath holds + 4–6 breathing for stress	Walk while repeating your Personal Power Affirmation aloud or silently, syncing it with your breath	Revisit the Two-Paths Visualization (as above)
13	Chapter 5	30- to 60-second cold shower	2 or 3 rounds Tummo breathing + affirmations during breath holds	Microcosmic Orbit Flow with Arm Movements	Journal about your Qi Gong experience (could you feel energy or Qi flow through your hands or body?)
14	Chapter 5	30- to 60-second cold shower	2 or 3 rounds Tummo breathing + affirmations during breath holds + 4–7–8 breathing before bed	Tai Chi Walk (or begin learning a Tai Chi form)	Journal about how your Tai Chi Walk felt: Were you able to stay present with each step and breath, or did your thoughts wander? Notice any changes in your mood, tension, or mental clarity

15	Chapter 5	60- to 120-second cold shower	2 or 3 rounds Tummo breathing + affirmations and mindfulness during breath holds outside	Practice a set of sun salutations followed by Yin Yoga (gentle stretching)	Reflect on your sun salutations. How did your body feel during the flow? Did your breath sync naturally with your movement?
16	Chapter 6	60- to 120-second cold shower	3 or 4 rounds Tummo breathing + affirmations during breath holds + 4–6 breathing when anxious	Walk while repeating your Personal Power Affirmation aloud or silently, syncing it with your breath	Journal how your walk felt (did the affirmation feel more powerful?)

| 17 | Chapter 6 | 60- to 120-second cold shower | 2-3 rounds Tummo breathing + affirmations and mindfulness during breath holds | Microcosmic Orbit Flow with Arm Movements | Craft a Pain-Pleasure Affirmation: Choose a habit you want to change, then write 3 bullet points describing the pain it causes you, and 3 describing the blessings you'll gain by letting it go. Then combine them into one powerful affirmation |

18	Chapter 6	60- 120-second cold shower	2 or 3 rounds Tummo breathing + affirmations during breath holds + 4–7–8 breathing before bed	Practice a set of sun salutations followed by Yin Yoga (gentle stretching)	Self-Forgiveness exercise: Identify moments of regret. Write down a list of past regrets, then write a compassionate reframe for each one—turning guilt into growth by acknowledging what you learned and how you've changed
19	Chapter 7	Optional cold plunge	2 or 3 rounds Tummo breathing + affirmations and mindfulness during breath holds	Yin Yoga/gentle stretching with intention-first thing in the morning	Morning Ritual: Design and follow a 4-part habit stack including breathwork, affirmation, hydration, and cold exposure

20	Chapter 7	60- to 120-second cold shower	3 or 4 rounds Tummo breathing + affirmations during breath holds right before cold shower	Yin Yoga/gentle stretching before bed	Evening Wind-Down: Journal about your screen-free time, and what helps you wind down effectively
21	Chapter 7	60- to 120-second cold shower	2 or 3 rounds Tummo breathing + affirmations and mindfulness during breath holds outside + 4–6 breathing when stressed	Mindful walk outside. Be present in your breath and body as you walk	See Who You're Becoming: Imagine yourself 6 months from now, thriving in a life built on strong, daily habits. See yourself waking up refreshed, eating nourishing food, and handling stress with ease

22	Chapter 8	Cold plunge or 2-minute shower	2 or 3 rounds Tummo breathing + affirmations during breath holds + evening 4–7–8	Walk while repeating your Personal Power Affirmation aloud or silently, syncing it with your breath	Create Your "no" script: Write and practice your response to an offer that could trigger relapse
23	Chapter 8	Cold plunge or 2-minute shower	2 or 3 rounds Tummo breathing + affirmations mindfulness during breath holds outside	Practice a set of sun salutations followed by Yin Yoga (gentle stretching)	Accountability Check-In: Journal how you'll seek support online or with a trusted person this week
24	Chapter 8	60- to 120-second cold shower	3 or 4 rounds Tummo breathing + affirmations during breath holds	Tai Chi Walk or begin learning a Tai Chi form	Revisit the Two-Paths Visualization (as above)
25	Chapter 9	60- to 120 second cold shower	2 or 3 rounds Tummo breathing + affirmations and mindfulness during breath holds	Walk outside, noticing how your values show up in the world around you	Core Values Exercise: Go through the list of values in Chapter 9 and pick 3 to 5 that resonate most

26	Chapter 9	60- to 120-second cold shower	2 or 3 rounds Tummo breathing + affirmations during breath holds +4–6 breathing before bed	Walk while repeating your "Why" Statement aloud or silently, syncing it with your breath	Write or revise your "Why" Statement based on your values and the life you want
27	Chapter 9	Cold plunge	3 to 5 rounds Tummo breathing + affirmations during breath holds	Step forward and backward physically while saying your old label and your new label	Label Liberation: Identify one limiting label and reframe it into an empowering one
28	Chapter 10	60- to 120-second cold shower or cold plunge	2 or 3 rounds Tummo breathing + affirmations and mindfulness during breath holds	Take one step toward practicing your identified passion, no matter how small, then reward yourself	Passion Snapshot: Identify one activity you want to try this week and why it excites you
29	Chapter 10	60- to 120-second cold shower	2 or 3 rounds Tummo breathing + affirmations during breath holds +4–7–8 breathing before bed	Walk while repeating your Personal Power Affirmation aloud or silently, syncing it with your breath	Tribe Building: List 5 ways to connect with like-minded people online or in person

30	Chapter 10	60- to 120-second cold shower or cold plunge	3 or 4 rounds Tummo breathing + affirmations during breath holds outside	Walk while repeating your "Why" Statement aloud or silently, syncing it with your breath	Revisit the Two-Paths Visualization (as above)

APPENDIX C: NOTES

References for the Introduction

1. Andrews, D., & Canfield, J. (2016). The 30-Day Sobriety Solution: How to Cut Back or Quit Drinking in the Privacy of Your Own Home. Atria Books.
2. Tang, Y.-Y., & Posner, M. I. (2015). The neuroscience of mindfulness meditation. *Nature Reviews Neuroscience, 16*(4), 213–225. https://doi.org/10.1038/nrn3916

References for Chapter 1

1. Koob, G. F., & Volkow, N. D. (2016). Neurobiology of addiction: A neurocircuitry analysis. The Lancet Psychiatry, 3(8), 760–773. https://doi.org/10.1016/S2215-0366(16)00104-8
2. National Institute on Alcohol Abuse and Alcoholism (NIAAA). (2022). Alcohol facts and statistics. https://www.niaaa.nih.gov/
3. Seo, D., & Sinha, R. (2015). Neuroplasticity and predictors of alcohol recovery. Alcohol Research: Current Reviews, 37(1), 143–152. https://www.ncbi.nlm.nih.gov/pmc/articles/PMC4476600/
4. World Health Organization. (2018). *Global status report on alcohol and health*. World Health Organization. https://www.who.int/publications/i/item/9789241565639

References for Chapter 2

1. Cohen, G. L., & Sherman, D. K. (2014). Cohen, G. L., & Sherman, D. K. (2014). *The psychology of change: Self-affirmation and social psychological intervention. Annual Review of Psychology*, 65, 333–371. https://doi.org/10.1146/annurev-psych-010213-115137

2. Dweck, C. S. (2006). Mindset: The new psychology of success. Random House.
3. Lembke, A. (2021). Dopamine Nation: Finding Balance in the Age of Indulgence. Dutton.
4. Volkow, N. D., Koob, G. F., & McLellan, A. T. (2016). Neurobiologic Advances from the Brain Disease Model of Addiction. The New England Journal of Medicine, 374(4), 363–371. https://doi.org/10.1056/NEJMra1511480

References for Chapter 3

1. Hopper, S. I., Murray, S. L., Ferrara, L. R., & Singleton, J. K. (2019). Effectiveness of diaphragmatic breathing for reducing physiological and psychological stress in adults: A quantitative systematic review. JBI Database of Systematic Reviews and Implementation Reports, 17(9), 1855–1876. https://doi.org/10.11124/JBISRIR-2017-003848
2. Perciavalle, V., Blandini, M., Fecarotta, P., Buscemi, A., Di Corrado, D., Bertolo, L., Fichera, F., & Coco, M. (2017). The role of deep breathing on stress. Neurological Sciences, 38(3), 451–458. https://doi.org/10.1007/s10072-016-2790-8

References for Chapter 4

1. Brown, R. P., & Gerbarg, P. L. (2009). Yoga breathing, meditation, and longevity. *Annals of the New York Academy of Sciences, 1172*, 54–62. https://doi.org/10.1111/j.1749-6632.2009.04394.x
2. Carney, S. (2017). What Doesn't Kill Us: How Freezing Water, Extreme Altitude, and Environmental Conditioning Will Renew Our Lost Evolutionary Strength. Rodale.
3. Kox, M., van Eijk, L. T., Zwaag, J., van den Wildenberg, J., Sweep, F. C. G. J., van der Hoeven, J. G., & Pickkers, P. (2014). Voluntary activation of the sympathetic nervous system and attenuation of the innate immune response in

humans. *PNAS, 111*(20), 7379–7384.
https://doi.org/10.1073/pnas.1322176111

4. Srámek, P., Simecková, M., Janský, L., Savlíková, J., & Vybíral, S. (2000). Human physiological responses to immersion into water of different temperatures. *European Journal of Applied Physiology*, 81(5), 436–442. https://doi.org/10.1007/s004210050065

5. van Marken Lichtenbelt, W. D., & Schrauwen, P. (2011). Impacts of cold exposure on energy expenditure and metabolism. *Trends in Endocrinology & Metabolism, 22*(11), 353–359. https://doi.org/10.1016/j.tem.2011.07.009

References for Chapter 5

1. Chen, X., Cui, J., Li, R., Norton, R., Park, J., Kong, J., & Yeung, A. (2019). Dao Yin (a.k.a. Qigong): Origin, development, potential mechanisms, and clinical applications. Evidence-Based Complementary and Alternative Medicine, 2019, 3705120. https://doi.org/10.1155/2019/3705120

2. Clear, J. (2018). Atomic Habits: An Easy & Proven Way to Build Good Habits & Break Bad Ones. Avery.

3. Csikszentmihalyi, M. (1990). *Flow: The Psychology of Optimal Experience*. Harper Perennial.

4. Liu, J., Shi, H., & Lee, T. M. C. (2023). Qigong exercise and cognitive function in brain imaging studies: A systematic review of randomized controlled trials in healthy and cognitively impaired populations. *NeuroImage: Clinical, 40*, 103345.

5. Robbins, A. (1991). *Awaken the Giant Within*. Free Press.

6. Tolle, E. (1997). The Power of Now: A Guide to Spiritual Enlightenment. Namaste Publishing.

7. Wayne, P. M., & Fuerst, M. L. (2013). Harvard Medical School Guide to Tai Chi: 12 Weeks to a Healthy Body, Strong Heart, and Sharp Mind. Shambhala Publications.

8. Zou, L., Sasaki, J. E., Wei, G. X., Huang, T., Yeung, A. S., Neto, O. B., Chen, K. W., & Hui, S. S. (2018). Effects of mind–body exercises (Tai Chi/Yoga) on heart rate variability parameters and perceived stress: A systematic review with meta-analysis of randomized controlled trials. *Journal of Clinical Medicine, 7*(11), 404. https://doi.org/10.3390/jcm7110404

References for Chapter 6

1. Beck, A. T., Wright, F. D., Newman, C. F., & Liese, B. S. (1994). *Cognitive Therapy of Substance Abuse.* Guilford Press.
2. Clear, J. (2018). Atomic Habits: An Easy & Proven Way to Build Good Habits & Break Bad Ones. Avery.
3. Dweck, C. S. (2006). *Mindset: The New Psychology of Success.* Ballantine Books.
4. Lembke, A. (2021). Dopamine Nation: Finding Balance in the Age of Indulgence. Dutton.
5. Lieberman, M. D., Eisenberger, N. I., Crockett, M. J., Tom, S. M., Pfeifer, J. H., & Way, B. M. (2007). Putting feelings into words: Affect labeling disrupts amygdala activity in response to affective stimuli. *Psychological Science, 18*(5), 421–428. https://doi.org/10.1111/j.1467-9280.2007.01916.x
6. Robbins, T. (1991). Awaken the Giant Within: How to Take Immediate Control of Your Mental, Emotional, Physical & Financial Destiny! Free Press.

References for Chapter 7

1. Clear, J. (2018). Atomic Habits: An Easy & Proven Way to Build Good Habits & Break Bad Ones. Avery.
2. Huberman, A. (2021). *Huberman Lab Podcast.* https://hubermanlab.com
3. Kabat-Zinn, J. (2013). Full Catastrophe Living: Using the Wisdom of Your Body and Mind to Face Stress, Pain, and Illness. (Revised ed.) Bantam Books.

4. Selhub, E. M. (2015). *Nutritional psychiatry: Your brain on food.* Harvard Health Publishing. Retrieved from https://www.health.harvard.edu/blog/nutritional-psychiatry-your-brain-on-food-201511168626

References for Chapter 8

1. Lembke, A. (2021). Dopamine Nation: Finding Balance in the Age of Indulgence. Dutton.
2. National Institute on Drug Abuse (NIDA). (2021). *Cannabis (Marijuana) Research Report.* https://nida.nih.gov

References for Chapter 9

1. Csikszentmihalyi, M. (1990). Flow: The Psychology of Optimal Experience. Harper & Row.
2. Dweck, C. S. (2006). Mindset: The New Psychology of Success. Ballantine Books.
3. Emmons, R. A., & McCullough, M. E. (2003). Counting blessings versus burdens: An experimental investigation of gratitude and subjective well-being in daily life. Journal of Personality and Social Psychology, 84(2), 377–389. https://doi.org/10.1037/0022-3514.84.2.377
4. Frankl, V. E. (1959). Man's Search for Meaning. Beacon Press.
5. Lin, W.-F., Mack, D., Enright, R. D., Krahn, D., & Baskin, T. W. (2004). Effects of forgiveness therapy on anger, mood, and vulnerability to substance use among inpatient substance-dependent clients. Journal of Consulting and Clinical Psychology, 72(6), 1114–1121. https://doi.org/10.1037/0022-006X.72.6.1114
6. Ryan, R. M., & Deci, E. L. (2017). Self-Determination Theory: Basic Psychological Needs in Motivation, Development, and Wellness. Guilford Press.
7. Tolle, E. (1997). *The Power of Now.* New World Library.

References for Chapter 10

1. Beattie, M. C., & Longabaugh, R. (1999). General and alcohol-specific social support following treatment. Journal of Substance Abuse Treatment, 17(1–2), 37–44.

2. Chekroud, S. R., Gueorguieva, R., Zheutlin, A. B., Paulus, M., Krumholz, H. M., Krystal, J. H., & Chekroud, A. M. (2018). Association between physical exercise and mental health in 1.2 million individuals in the USA between 2011 and 2015: a cross-sectional study. *The Lancet Psychiatry, 5*(9), 739–746. https://doi.org/10.1016/S2215-0366(18)30227-X

3. Clear, J. (2018). Atomic Habits: An Easy & Proven Way to Build Good Habits & Break Bad Ones. Avery.

4. Csikszentmihalyi, M. (1990). *Flow: The Psychology of Optimal Experience*. Harper & Row.

5. Lembke, A. (2021). Dopamine Nation: Finding Balance in the Age of Indulgence. Dutton.

www.ingramcontent.com/pod-product-compliance
Lightning Source LLC
Chambersburg PA
CBHW031620040426
42452CB00007B/592